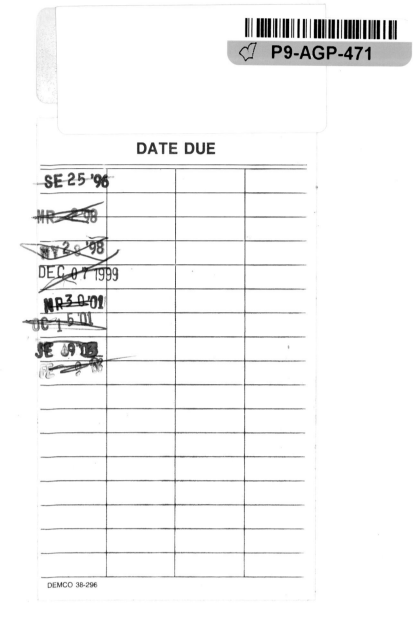

P9-AGP-471

DATE DUE

SE 25 '96		
MR 2 '98		
MY 2 8 '98		
DEC 0 7 1999		
MR 3 0 '01		
OC 1 5 '01		
SE 09 '03		
FE 2 '08		

DEMCO 38-296

Viropause/Andropause
The Male Menopause

Viropause/ Andropause

The Male Menopause

Emotional and Physical Changes Mid-Life Men Experience

Dr. Aubrey M. Hill

NEW HORIZON PRESS
Far Hills, New Jersey

Requests for permission should be addressed to:
New Horizon Press
P.O. Box 669
Far Hills, NJ 07931

Hill, Aubrey M.
      Viropause/Andropause: The male menopause. Emotional and physical changes mid-life men experience.

Library of Congress Catalog Card Number: 93-84520

ISBN: 0-88282-084-2 (hc)
          0-88282-080-X (pb)
New Horizon Press

Manufactured in the U.S.A.

1997 1996 1995 1994 1993 / 5 4 3 2 1

Dedication

To my best teachers, my patients

Contents

CONTENTS

Author's Note

Readers will find that many of the topics in this book are addressed to men who are presumably married. This is merely a convenience and is not meant to imply that the material presented does not apply to single men or to men in other types of relationships. I found it more convenient to refer to a wife rather than list, each time it was appropriate, such words as *partner, consort, associate, companion,* or *lover.*

Male menopause is a condition that affects both married and single men, heterosexual and homosexual men. I find nothing in the scientific literature to suggest that any man, regardless of orientation or relational status, is immune to the viropause/andropause syndrome. However, there is no information available on the relative incidence of male menopause among these different relational populations of men. In my own practice, I have observed no differences in the incidence of male menopause among the various populations of men.

This book is based on my professional experience.

However, the patients and individuals mentioned in this book are not specific individuals but composites, and all names are ficticious.

Acknowledgments

I wish to acknowledge and to thank the following.

Esther Hill, my wife, who listened to me read the first drafts, offered helpful comments and suggestions, and gave me much encouragement; Carolyn Crowley, B.S., who proofread the text and made many helpful editorial contributions; Helen Clough, my secretary, who typed the original manuscript, handled the mailing, kept the books, and learned a new computer system to help me finish the book; Natasha Kern, my agent, who believed in the project from the start despite its controversial nature; Alice Price Knight, Professional Writing Services in Denver, who took my original manuscript, reorganized the chapters, and rewrote it so it would be comprehensible and acceptable to the publisher; Mike Hepworth, Department of Sociology, University of Aberdeen, UK, who assessed the subject matter, made helpful recommendations, offered encouragement, and arranged contacts with other writers in the UK; Ronald Taylor, Ph.D., clinical psychologist, who reviewed the manuscript and made suggestions about improving it;

ACKNOWLEDGMENTS

David Kirkpatrick, M.D., psychiatrist, who gave good advice and made important contributions to the manuscript; Don Skillman, a patient, a friend, and a writer of books, who gave me invaluable advice on writing and on the intricacies of book publishing; Jeanette Friedli, M.D., psychiatrist in Zurich, Switzerland, who interviewed psychiatrists in continental Europe for me and provided valuable information during my research into the subject of andropause; my colleagues, Arthur Burnett, M.D., Johns Hopkins University School of Medicine, and Eric Orwall, M.D., Oregon Health Sciences University, who gave of their time and expertise on various facets of male menopause.

Introduction

Many of my male patients who are in their forties and fifties have come to see me over the years with amazingly similar symptoms. At first, I did not regard their physical symptoms as being related to their age, but after numerous cases, I began to suspect that there was a connection. Though these men usually have physical complaints, some of their symptoms are frequently the result of psychological and emotional difficulties that stem from natural mid-life changes.

My medical training had not prepared me for finding a connection between men's physical symptoms and the period of life in which they occur. When I searched the medical literature for information about mid-life changes in men, I found almost nothing on the subject. Medical science has been conspicuously silent about the changes that I see men commonly experiencing during mid-life.

Although the physical changes are generally not medical crises, many men experience them as traumatic. I believe the trauma results, in part, from the fact that most men know so little about what changes to expect in their bodies in mid-life. Not knowing what to expect, they frequently fear the worst.

Research into male mid-life changes has only recently been initiated. In marked contrast, there has been much research into the changes that occur in women in mid-life. As a result, the physical and mental changes of female menopause are well understood. I might speculate about the reasons for this disparity in information, but whatever the reasons, the lack of scientific data about the physical and psychological changes of middle-aged men is a situation that needs to be corrected.

Though I did not believe it at the outset, my experience has now convinced me that most men undergo what could be called male menopause and that many men suffer acutely and needlessly because they don't have access to the information they need to understand their symptoms.

Not all men are adversely affected by the changes that occur in middle age, but many are. Some become seriously depressed, or get caught up in negative behavior patterns that impede their ability to transcend the emotional difficulties they experience at this stage of their lives. They may become extremely unhappy and feel hopeless about the future. They are unable to believe that fulfillment and happiness can lie ahead. They think that the best of life is over.

The first step in coping with male menopause is to recognize that it exists. With so little medical literature on the subject, it hasn't been easy to accept male menopause as real. Even now, there is little medical information available about the sexual and mental changes men can normally expect, and what exists is often considered controversial.

This book is not intended as a political tract but rather

as a medical exploration of previously unpublicized information. To suggest that men may suffer difficult physical and emotional transitions in mid-life is in no way meant to dismiss or diminish the different transitions women experience in menopause. Increased knowledge can bring increased understanding.

More people are reaching middle age than ever before, and the need for information is greater than ever. Not only are the numbers of the middle-aged men increasing, but their expectations are changing as well. Men want more for themselves in the years after middle age than their fathers might have. They want to know that they can anticipate a continuing sense of fulfillment and happiness as they age, not just resignation. They don't want to believe, as our culture often seems to insist, that being young is everything and that the loss of youth means the loss of virility, of happiness, and of productivity. They want to continue to enjoy life.

But if men are afraid to let go of their youth, they will not be able to make the transition to the next stage of life. If they can't believe that life in the middle years and in old age offers its own contentments and joys, how will they be able to go forward? Of the Biblical "four score years and ten" that men are allotted, it is not only the first forty that have a potential for growth and happiness. Though we tend to think of adulthood as one seamless fabric from adolescence to old age, it is not. There are within it recognizable stages that have only recently been identified, and whose significance is only beginning to be understood.

What I have learned from my patients about the male menopause may help others understand what it is and how to deal with it. I decided to write this book because it is apparent that men, not just women, experience physical and emotional mid-life changes. I hope more information on the subject can allay some of the anxiety so many men, and their wives or companions, feel about the coming years.

It is my further hope that this book will help men, and women as well, to recognize the male menopause as a potential source of difficulties men experience in their lives, help them to understand the changes, and help them to learn how they can effectively deal with male menopause.

CHAPTER 1

Men, Menopause, and Viropause/Andropause

Most of us think that only women experience an acute physical and emotional transition in middle age: the menopause. But men, too, experience physical and emotional changes in their middle years that involve more than the conventional mid-life crisis, changes that can seriously disrupt their lives and the lives of those who are close to them.

As they enter middle age, many men become concerned about the slight decrease they perceive in their sexuality. Actually, these are usually small changes in erectile firmness, delay of orgasm, and libido reduction, but they can cause enormous anxiety. Psychological changes that occur in mid-life can be disturbing enough to interfere with a man's mental and physical health. These symptoms can affect his ability to function as a marriage partner, lover, or father, and they can impair his performance at work.

Fifteen men in a hundred will experience symptoms severe enough that they could be considered to be suffering from an illness. However, only a small portion of those affected will consult a medical doctor or mental health professional for treatment of their symptoms. The other eighty-five percent of American men may not be diagnosed as ill, but their mid-life changes can cause serious problems that, for some, are long-lasting. Though the symptoms are classified as a medical entity, as is women's menopause, it does not mean that they represent an illnes per se. Rather, they are part of the viropause/andropause syndrome that, like puberty or menopause, is a naturally occuring life stage.

The phrase *mid-life crisis* is familiar to most people, and it is useful because it helps make both men and women aware that they need to adjust to the changes that occur in their lives and in their bodies as they age. Although andropause and the mid-life crisis have some similarities, they are not the same. While mid-life crisis refers to a passing philosophical life phase, the term *andropause* is more restrictive and limited in its use in describing a distinct medical entity. Andropause is a medical syndrome, an illness with a complex of symptoms, some of which may require medical or psychological treatment.

For men, there is no parallel to the physical stoppage a woman goes through when her hormones decrease and her periods end. The physical changes men experience vary considerably from man to man. The psychological andropausal symptoms are frequently accompanied by physical problems, sometimes psychosomatic ones, that cause the sufferer to seek medical help. Unfortunately, few doctors are able to provide that help because, until recently, medical information about male mid-life changes was not readily available to physicians.

Today the most common term used to identify the syndrome of changes is *male menopause*, but that expression can be misleading because the root of the word, *meno*, comes from the Greek word *menses*, and it refers to the female's monthly menstrual cycle. The *pause* or stopping of that cycle is menopause, and it is the major physical change that occurs in a woman in mid-life. One term for the male transitional experience is *andropause*, a term used in Europe but not yet generally familiar to American readers, although it has been used in the medical literature since 1975. The root of *andropause* is *andro*, which is Greek for man. Recently, the synonym *viropause* has been used on television and in magazines. *Vir* is the Latin prefix for man. Both terms may be used interchangeably with *male menopause* and are useful as a way to acknowledge the similarities of the aging processes in men and women. Many of us in the medical profession have begun to recognize that much of the aging experience of the two sexes is similar.

Mid-Life Changes

More men are reaching middle age than at any time in history; their expectations are changing, and the need for information is greater than ever. Men want more for themselves in the years after middle age than their fathers had. They want to know that they can anticipate happiness, fulfillment, and sexual satisfaction, not just retirement. They don't want to believe, as our culture seems to insist, that being young is everything.

Middle-aged men with hair pieces, wearing gold chains, driving hot red sports cars, and divorcing their wives to marry sexy women young enough to be their daughters are an integral part of our cultural mythology. We all laugh when we see a character portrayed this way—such as the Joe Pesci character in the *Lethal Weapon* movies. We laugh because we recognize the type—we all know a man who, when he hit his forties, suddenly seemed to lose all of his common sense.

All of us eventually, and sometimes painfully, arrive at the realization that youth does not last. In middle life, we need to redefine our purpose and reshape our identity if we are to find happiness in our later years. This redefining and reshaping is the special task of this time in our lives. The symptoms of menopause compel all of us of either gender to take on that task.

In her middle years, a woman's monthly cycle comes to an end along with her ability to reproduce. The alterations in hormones that bring about the end of the menstrual cycle are also related to other changes in her body and frequently affect her emotional state.

As women enter menopause, their hormone levels change as their production of estrogen slows, a change that can be verified through laboratory tests. The decrease in estrogen produces several definite physical symptoms. One of these is the irregularity and eventual end of monthly periods. Another change affects the system that regulates body temperature—the body's thermostat, so to speak. The result is the "hot flashes" that many women experience during menopause.

For men, changes in hormones are gradual and not as easy to confirm in laboratory tests. However, for many men the sexual and physical changes do occur, though they may vary somewhat from man to man. Psychological changes that occur in mid-life can be disturbing enough to interfere with the man's mental or physical health.

Though sexual activity may gradually decline during middle age, only rarely is there any physical reason for men to lose their sexual potency. They remain fertile, usually well into old age. Still, virility seems to concern men most.

"Most men approaching middle age become concerned over sexual performance," says author Miriam Stoppard in her book *50-Plus Life Guide,* in which she equates increasing anxiety over sexuality with male menopause. Men frequently come to my office because they have become aware of a decreased interest in sex and are worried about it or have difficulty in performing sexually as frequently or as vigorously as they used to. However, when I ask them questions, their answers frequently reveal that their concern about their sexuality are just the tip of the iceberg. With supportive questioning, they often reveal other deep dissatisfactions with their lives. They are happy to learn that their condition is not unique and that the consequences of aging are not as threatening as they might appear to be. Men in middle age need to be reassured that their masculinity is intact and that the years ahead offer the possibility of increased fulfillment and a probability of deepened joy in their lives once they are past the transition point of male menopause. But simply talking about it is seldom enough.

Often, men of forty or so come to see me because of insomnia, or because they are suffering from an unaccustomed sense of fatigue. Though insomnia and sexual difficulties may seem to have little in common, I have found that the concerns of middle-aged insomnia patients are remarkably similar to the concerns of those worried about their sexuality. These two physical manifestations—sexual problems and sleep problems—are the most commonly occurring outward symptoms of the inner turmoil that men experience in their middle years. This turmoil has its origins in an awareness, conscious or unconscious, of the aging of their bodies.

Recent Studies of Andropause

For years, male aging received so little attention that most medical professionals did not acknowledge it as a problem. Only in the last two decades has medical science begun to study the changes that men undergo. In contrast, the climacteric—the medical term for mid-life change in women—has been studied extensively for almost seventy years. In fact, laboratory analysis of female hormone changes occurring with age goes back to 1925. In 1938, estrogen agents first became available.

Though it has taken almost fifty years, the male menopause has begun to be recognized as a potential cause of physical and emotional problems. The terms *male menopause, male climacteric, viropause,* and *andropause* have begun to appear in the medical literature. With this recent scrutiny, medical researchers have identified a distinct complex of symptoms associated with the male menopause.

Though the increase in information about male aging has been rapid, medical articles dealing with the problems of aging in women still outnumber those about aging in men by a hundred to one. There are many reasons for the unequal attention paid to male and female mid-life changes. One is that many of the symptoms of male menopause tend to be more psychological and thus more difficult to analyze and define than are conditions that are primarily physical. There are no easily identifiable changes in a man's reproductive system that correspond to the end of a woman's monthly menstrual cycle. Another reason is that andropausal symptoms can vary greatly while women in menopause have a number of symptoms in common like hot flashes, mood changes, and irregularity. For men, except for mood changes, there are no typical symptoms. The male syndrome of mid-life is not easy to describe. Laboratory procedures are of little assistance in confirming or ruling out the presence of menopause in men.

Diagnosing Andropause

The male climacteric can occur without producing any distinct medical problems. But for women, the loss of estrogen can have medical consequences. For example, loss of estrogen accelerates osteoporosis, the diminishing of bone density. This can increase a woman's susceptibility to bone fractures as well as other painful skeletal changes. Because their hormones are different, men are less likely to suffer from osteoporosis.

The term *mid-life crisis* encompasses a wide variety of symptoms common to both men and women in their middle years. Although the viropause/andropause syndrome and mid-life crisis have important similarities, they are not the same. The term *andropause* is more restrictive and limited in its use. It describes a distinct medical entity, a syndrome with a complex of symptoms that may require medical or psychological treatment. Viropause/andropause does not simply refer to a phase of life, as does the term *mid-life crisis*. As the proportion of our population in their middle years increases, the need to understand their particular problems is becoming more important. Because viropause is a syndrome and not a passing phase of an individual's life, we need to understand how it can be effectively diagnosed and treated.

A patient of mine, Kyle Beldere, was returning from a business trip three weeks before his fifty-second birthday when he became vaguely uncomfortable with thoughts of returning home. He recalled how he had felt just a year or two before, how he would anticipate walking through the door into the arms of his wife and talk about the happenings of the trip. But now the prospect did not excite him, and he almost dreaded his arriving. This had been a successful trip, his marketing proposals had been received with enthusiasm, but the thought of returning to the office saddened him. Only a year before he would have been eager to start a new week with its challenges.

Kyle had expected his home life to take a new and happier turn when his youngest daughter left for college, but instead the quiet routine became a bit boring. Watching his wife toweling after her shower did not stimulate him as it had before. For the first time in his life, he had misgivings about his sexuality and masculinity.

A friend of Kyle's suggested a holiday, so two weeks later he and his wife went to the friend's mountain cabin. It was a secluded, pleasant place. No one else was within shouting distance. On the drive up, Kyle started to relax and become more aware of his surroundings.

After arriving, Kyle split wood while his wife stored the groceries. The physical exertion of swinging the ax felt good, and he recalled the pleasures of physically productive work he had experienced as a teenager. They had lunch on the deck in the autumn sun, read, and totally forgot the outside world.

For most of their married lives, holidays and weekends were spent with others and were often hectic. They were fun, but left little time for closeness. On this peaceful weekend, it seemed natural to spend more time in the physical expression of love. The usual pattern of their lovemaking was twenty to thirty minutes duration and often when one or both were tired. This time they were both relaxed and were more aware of their closeness. Much of the next day, also, was spent in lovemaking. On the way home, Kyle realized that he was now quietly pleased with his sexuality.

During mid-life, libido decreases somewhat, but doesn't disappear. Erectile and orgasmic functions also change, but are certainly adequate for pleasurable, loving, and very satisfying intercourse.

Being concerned about his afternoon lethargy at work, Kyle arranged an appointment with me. The exam and tests showed no significant abnormalities, but I offered some advice regarding a change in health habits for middle age.

Kyle discontinued having wine with lunch and reduced his food intake for this meal. His new lunch consisted of a salad, light on the dressing, and a roll. Almost immediately he regained his afternoon stamina. He reduced his coffee intake to two cups in the morning and none after the ten o'clock break. He limited his alcohol to one cocktail before dinner or one glass of wine with the meal. After changing his coffee and alcohol habits, he noticed his sleeping pattern improved. He fell asleep promptly upon retiring, slept well through the night, and felt refreshed in the morning. He no longer required four cups of coffee to come up to speed in the morning or a caffeine fix at intervals during the work day.

Some people can drink coffee throughout the day and sleep well. Others develop a sensitivity to the caffeine which results in restless, non-restorative sleep. The morning caffeine improves wakefulness but has a delayed withdrawal effect of restlessness or irritability several hours later.

Alcohol in the evening may result in falling asleep promptly, but causes restless sleep in the last half of the night. When taken in larger amounts, alcohol causes the drinker to waken after two to four hours and then he is often unable to return to sleep.

I also suggested some changes in Kyle's exercise program. He discontinued his daily four-mile run and substituted fast-walking a mile each way to and from work. He also started walking briskly between shots on the golf course instead of riding a cart. These changes reduced the occasional muscle and joint strain he had been experiencing from the running. He missed the euphoria of the running and disliked the diminished self-image of not being a runner, but the absence of the pain and a sustained feeling of well-being made it worthwhile.

Aerobic exercise is to be encouraged, and most middle-aged adults can exercise vigorously without damage to their skeletal system. However, the type and amount of exercise should be individualized. For some, the pounding trauma of running can exacerbate earlier injuries and hasten the onset of arthritis.

Kyle's golfing partner, Al, never wore a hat on the links. One day he found a darkened spot on the back of his neck which, when removed, was diagnosed as melanoma. Despite surgery and other treatments, the cancer spread. The condition progressed rapidly and Al died eight months after some new tumors appeared.

During these eight months, Al and Kyle had many serious conversations. One afternoon after returning from a round of golf and conversation with Al, Kyle became aware of a vague feeling of depression. As he analyzed this feeling, he suddenly realized that he had been forced to think about his own mortality.

Subsequent talks with Al became more intense. Al told

of his changing values and priorities. The support from his family and friends became increasingly important to him. He was somewhat surprised to learn that, while they appreciated his occupational and financial success, they respected him more as a person for his honesty and caring and appreciation of the beauty in the world around him.

Kyle started relating Al's observations to his own life. He reassessed the relative importance of status and financial success to the importance of his interpersonal relationships. His wife's years of love and caring were reappraised. Even though he loved her and appreciated her love, he had never given it deep thought. He became more acutely aware of her concerns for him and became more tolerant of her habits that had previously irritated him.

Though Kyle would not have expressed it this way, he matured. Unfortunately, it took the terminal illness of a good friend to make his introspections possible.

For several weeks, Kyle progressed through the usual stages of grieving for Al. By the time he reached the acceptance stage, thoughts of his own eventual death became pervasive.

Fear of death can be overwhelming in some men and even cause viropausal/andropausal symptoms. A healthy mental adjustment to mid-life is an essential element to recovery.

Kyle's first and most painful step was to acknowledge that he too would die some day. After that, he derived some comfort from thinking about the many good years still left, about the happy memories he would be leaving with his wife and friends, and about the possibility of awareness after death or the escape it would provide from discomfort and unhappiness.

Even thought Kyle was healthy and still "too young to die," he consulted an attorney and drew up a will. He was surprised to discover how painless the process was. Preparing and filing a will removes a source of anxiety and reduces the fear of death. It forced Kyle to think more realistically about dying and to make some adjustments to his views about the termination of experiences.

By Kyle's fifty-fourth birthday, he was both happier and more content. He felt at peace with himself and with others in his life and was again finding satisfaction in his work.

For the great majority of men . . . this period [middle age] evokes tumultuous struggles with the self and with the external world. Their midlife transistor is a time of moderate to severe crisis. Every aspect of their lives comes into question, and they are horrified by much that is revealed. They are full of recrimination against themselves and others. They cannot go on as before, but need time to choose a new path or modify the old one.

—Daniel J. Levinson,
The Seasons of a Man's Life

Kyle's experiences illustrate some of the typical concerns and anxieties that men experiencing male menopause face. More remedies for these and other concerns follow, as well as suggestions for both self-help and professional help to make the passage through viropause easier.

CHAPTER 2

Common Physical and Psychological Changes

Aging starts at the time of conception, but the negative aspects of aging don't begin until the fourth and fifth decades of life. Young people see themselves as indestructible and have little appreciation of their mortality. This attitude changes drastically in later life. Suddenly we become aware that we are growing old. For many people, each gray hair or perceived wrinkle becomes a matter of concern, and this is especially true of the man experiencing viropause.

The aging process has many intertwined causes, but the most prominent one, underlying all the rest, is the normal deterioration of the circulatory system. Every cell, organ, and body system needs a good blood supply to bring it oxygen and nutrients. As the efficiency of circulation decreases, deterioration (aging) occurs.

Continued decreased circulation is responsible for many of the physical and mental "symptoms" we associate with aging. The retina of the eye deteriorates when arteries fail to supply a good blood flow, and this impairs vision. Decreased circulation to the brain reduces mental acuity and memory. Heart muscles weaken and can fail from slowed circulation, although damaged arteries are more often responsible for heart attacks. A good blood supply is also needed to produce penile tumescence (erection), and many physical factors cause this blood supply to diminish in some men over fifty. And if the blood supply to the testes is blocked, atrophy occurs and testosterone production fails. Impaired circulation, along with ultraviolet exposure from the sun, is also responsible for aging of the skin: loss of tone, wrinkling, thinning, and discoloration. The effect is increased in those who use tobacco. Smoking also impairs blood flow to the penis and can be a cause of male impotence.

Recent research suggests that free radicals in the blood, byproducts of metabolism that damage protein enzymes, contribute to such aging processes as cataracts, memory impairment, and cardiovascular disease.

Some organs, such as the liver, have their evolution wired in. The liver undergoes a gradual reduction in function over time. Fortunately, this organ has a tremendous reserve of functioning cells so it's rarely a significant problem except for those having cirrhosis from excessive drinking.

Normal wear and tear over the years also causes changes most commonly seen in the weight-bearing joints such as the knees, hips, and lower back.

Physical Aging

Young men usually recover quickly and completely from sprains and strains with no residual discomfort or disability. Older men may not recover completely from injury and usually are more susceptible to re-injury. The realization that our bodies are letting us down—that we can't physically do what we used to do easily—can be a devastating one. Acknowledging that our physical deterioration, our signs of aging, are irreversible is often destructive to the self-image we developed when we were young.

For instance, during people's forties and fifties, normal skin undergoes several changes as pre-existing wrinkles deepen and elongate and new wrinkles appear. The reason is a loss of collagen (protein fibers), isolated fat deposits, and a reduction in tone of the underlying muscles. Foreheads wrinkle, bags enlarge under the eyes, and wattles appear under the chin. Muscle tone (normal tension), volume and strength decrease. Our muscles decrease in size and strength, although this is often reversible with appropriate exercise. The shape of the buttock changes, and wrinkles may develop between the buttocks and the back of the thighs. Depending on general body condition, weakened muscles may lower our endurance for physical activity. This is often described as a low energy level.

A receding hairline or graying or thinning hair are usually among the earliest signs of aging. Hereditary influences play a strong role in the timing and distribution of hair loss. The advertising and entertainment industries have turned the un-grayed, full head of hair into a symbol of youth, vitality, and masculinity. Despite our fascination with these icons, most graying or balding men make a good mental adjustment to these changes—but viropausal men do not.

During mid-life, people who have had normal vision often experience difficulty in reading small print. "I can't read the phone numbers unless there's a strong light" is one common complaint. This is called presbyopia. It is usually first noticed around the age of forty-five and often becomes a significant nuisance by age fifty. Magnifying eyeglasses can solve the problem, but the viropausal/andropausal male sees the need for glasses as one more depressing sign of his body's deterioration.

An important aspect of viropause is the physical changes in the body that accompany aging, including the reduction in sex drive. These changes leave a man with a sense of loss, feeling not just older but less masculine. And the physical changes can affect his emotions. He may feel a diminished sense of the importance or usefulness in his work and be unable to reflect on his future with his former confidence. Even though the physical changes are likely to be small and gradual, to the viropausal/andropausal man they have exaggerated importance. He may worry about the loss of his strength and his virility. (See Chapter 3 for more information on changes in sexuality).

Mental Aging

During our fifties and sixties, all of us experience some weakening of our mental sharpness, though the degree of this varies from person to person. This natural mental deterioration is recognized by the retirement conditions set out for many professions and industries. Airline pilots, for example, are retired at quite a young age because of the decline in their reflexes and mental acuity. Mandatory retirement for many occupations reflects society's awareness that the level of mental sharpness declines for those late in their middle years. In other areas this reduction is not as important. However, even a slight reduction can be troublesome to some people, especially to men experiencing male menopause.

Forgetfulness tops the list of mental changes in later life. Memory loss consistently occurs in older people as a natural symptom of aging (and should not be confused with Alzheimer's, which is a disease and not a natural process). We forget many things throughout our lives, but we usually ignore forgetfulness until we're older. Then, we tend to become more aware of it and see it as evidence that we are growing old. Additional symptoms people experience may be indecisiveness or impairment of the ability to reason carefully and make good decisions, especially decisions about the future.

The fact that our mental processes are slowing can become apparent in a variety of ways. It may take us longer to make decisions. For instance, we may have more trouble deciding which route to follow when planning a trip. Clarity of thought can also be reduced as irrelevant matters disrupt our normal progression of thought. Thought progression can be less orderly and intense concentration more difficult to achieve as distractions become more frequent and troublesome.

We all experience mental fatigue as the day progresses, but as we grow older, we can experience such tiredness with more profound effects. Unlike physical tiredness, which may feel good, mental fatigue produces feelings of listlessness, a low energy level, drowsiness, and sometimes irritability. A man experiencing male menopause obsesses over how tired he feels and is so troubled by it that he often becomes an annoyance to others.

CHAPTER 2

Dysphoria

Almost invariably, one of the symptoms of the viro-pause/andropause syndrome is a generalized sense of ill-being or of discontent. Doctors refer to such an emotional state as dysphoria, a term derived from the Greek word *dysphorous,* meaning hard to bear. Dysphoria can be described as agitation, excessive psychological pain, or anguish. Medically, it is defined as disquiet, restlessness, and malaise.

Dysphoria can take many different forms. The clearest way to explain this symptom is to say that the person who suffers from it is simply not a happy person. Though he may not actually describe himself as unhappy, he is not capable of feeling the sense of joy or satisfaction that he previously felt in his life.

During his annual physical exam, Victor Robertson, a patient of mine age forty-seven, told me in confidence that for the past several months he had been feeling depressed. Victor used the word *depressed*, as most people do, to indicate that he was unhappy. In medical terms, depression refers to a group of symptoms that include listlessness, withdrawal, changes in sleeping and eating patterns, despair, and reduced mental acuity, in addition to unhappiness. Victor's responses to my further questions did not indicate to me that he was clinically depressed.

As we talked about what was going on in his life and any changes that had occured since his last visit, Victor told me that the management of the company he worked for had changed and he was not enjoying his work as much as he used to. A few minutes later, he turned to another subject and asked me, "How are things with you and your wife now that your kids are in college?" After answering his question, I asked him in return, "How about you? Both your girls have moved out; how are you and your wife adjusting?"

He sighed. "I thought as soon as the kids were gone we'd have a lot more freedom and be happier, but it hasn't worked out that way." This admission opened a floodgate about his inexplicable feelings of unhappiness. He described his life as disenchanted. Various efforts to recapture the "joy of youth" had failed. His wife's suggestion that he needed a new hobby only annoyed him. Every thought of developing new interests seemed dull and even overwhelming.

Victor listened intently as I told him about the virpoause/andropause syndrome and how common his feelings were. He was relieved to learn he was not "losing it," but that there was a medical explanation for his gloomy feelings. I outlined a program to him for easing his negative feelings and coping with male menopause. He agreed to follow my suggestions but smiling asked, "Don't you have a pill that would fix things right now?" I shook my head, smiling in return. "I'd be a very rich doctor if I could invent a pill to reverse the natural aging process."

When a man in his forties or early fifties comes into the doctor's office with no definite symptoms, no specific complaints, and no easily discernible reason for seeking medical help, viropause may be the reason. If asked directly, "Are you enjoying life as much as you did a year or two ago?" he will usually respond with a negative answer. Often he will take several moments to reflect. Then he may typically concede, "No, I guess I'm not," and may volunteer an explanation. If he doesn't, questions may prompt him to elaborate. He may say, "I don't enjoy bowling as much as I used to." (Golf could be substituted here, or any number of physical activities from which he previously got pleasure.) "I've lost interest in club meetings," he may say, or "they don't make good movies like they used to, so I don't like to go any more," or "I used to enjoy my job, but now I almost dread going to work," or "I find the news boring these days." He may admit, "Even sex doesn't turn me on." Listening to him describe his feelings, it becomes all too clear that his life has lost its savor. Happiness is gone, and the unspoken concerns are "Why has it gone?" and "Has it gone for good?"

For the man experiencing it, this unhappiness is profound. It's not just a feeling of boredom or listlessness, it's disabling and lasts days or even weeks. The dysphoric person is preoccupied with unhappy thoughts which shut out productive thinking. Unpleasant events take on monumental importance and good things produce no joy or happiness. Most conversations deteriorate into morbid discussions. The dysphoric is a "glass is half empty" man.

It's unpleasant for others to be around him. He cannot be cheered up. A wife who tries frequently may give up and withdraw in anger. Employers and colleagues soon become aware of the dysphoric man's stormy mood and tend to avoid him. "Upbeat" employees are productive but the dysphoric's productivity declines. As his relationships deteriorate further, his problems intensify.

Alcohol and recreational drugs can create a feeling of euphoria, the opposite of dysphoria, so it's not surprising that viropausal men often use alcohol and drugs to treat their unhappiness. However, "coming down" and hangovers are similar in feeling to dysphoria so each down requires another drink or fix to alleviate the misery. The resulting vicious cycle can end in addiction.

Though some men who experience these anguished feelings of dysphoria do consult their doctors, a great many of them do not. There are several reasons that they don't. Some men don't really know that something is bothering them. Men are often not aware of their feelings on a conscious level. From childhood they are not encouraged to be aware of their feelings, and do not know how to describe them. It is also true that men are not expected to need help and find it difficult to seek it. The idea persists that it is somehow more masculine to suffer silently than to admit that something is wrong. Some men do not have much confidence that anyone can help them. They are used to thinking of themselves as strong and don't easily allow themselves to rely on others. Some men hesitate, partly because of masculine pride, to admit that they have feelings of unease or distress. There are other explanations as well, which, like these, may have their origins in the nature of our society and the ideas we all have about what is appropriate masculine and feminine behavior.

Anxiety

When a man experiences male menopause, he has uncertainty about his self-worth and is confused about priorities; therefore, there is anxiety. When there is anxiety he is apt to make major decisions for the wrong reasons.

Anxiety is frequently the emotional reaction to a sense of failure, of not having achieved expected goals. A man, as he approaches middle age, may compare what he has accomplished to that which he expected to accomplish in his youth and be discouraged. If he is asked, "What important goals do you have?" or "What do you intend to do with the rest of your life?" he may respond vaguely and evasively. Often the vagueness and evasion is in marked contrast to his previous self-confidence and ambition. Male menopause seems to affect most acutely those men who have had a particularly strong sense of purpose and personal drive. These are the men who are likely to become anxious and uncertain about the value of their achievements when they detect signs of aging and suddenly realize that their time is growing shorter.

Though anxiety is usually present in the viropause/andropause syndrome, that anxiety may not be apparent to the individual himself. To his family, his friends, or his colleagues at work, however, it becomes obvious. They may notice that he is irritable, cranky, short-tempered, or cross when previously he was not. Or they may see him as unusually quiet and withdrawn. Mood changes such as these are signs of the male menopause.

Men suffering from anxiety will sometimes describe themselves as restless or unaccountably nervous. Such a person may say to his doctor or someone else in whom he has chosen to confide, "I don't know what's the matter, but I feel shaky inside." He may demonstrate his shakiness by holding out a hand to show that it has a tremor. Though these individuals may know how they feel, they are probably at a loss to explain the cause. The search for a cause and a cure may bring them to seek help.

Often men who experience this anxiety have trouble sleeping. In fact, insomnia is often the "presenting symptom," the symptom that brings a patient to his doctor for help. A man in his forties or fifties who is otherwise healthy but has difficulty falling asleep or awakens during the night and is unable to return to sleep could be suffering from male menopause.

Sometimes insomnia is a part of a drinking problem. If a man drinks too much alcohol in the evening, telling himself that it will allow him to relax, he may fall asleep promptly when he retires, but then awaken later and be unable to return to sleep. Taking sedatives can produce other problems. When they are used at night, listlessness, depression, or both commonly occur during the day. The man can find himself between a rock and a hard place, choosing between insomnia and sedation. Insomnia can produce a daytime drowsiness or lack of energy and a feeling of being abnormally tired. In short, the anxiety that is a symptom of andropause frequently causes some form of sleep disorder or fatigue.

Anxiety can produce other symptoms as well. It can, for example, cause a variety of psychosomatic conditions such as headaches, indigestion, muscle aches and nervousness complaints. The fact that the mind affects the body is well known. Physical symptoms can have their origin in an individual's emotional state. Sometimes one or more of these symptoms will cause men to see a doctor. When no physical cause can be discovered and if these men are approaching middle age, it is reasonable to consider the possibility that the problem may be male menopause.

The man experiencing a menopausal discontent often develops anxiety in addition to his dysphoria. He is a nervous, unhappy person and may develop other physical conditions that have their origin in anxiety. Anxiety can also be caused by worrying, health problems, financial concerns, even the evening news. But regardless of source, anxiety often produces psychosomatic symptoms.

Headaches are a common complaint. Most headaches

are a response to tightening of muscles between the scalp and the skull or of the posterior neck. During anxiety, many people subconsciously tighten these muscles. There also seems to be a psychosomatic element for some migraine sufferers.

Stomach problems often develop. The gastrointestinal system is especially susceptible to the effects of the mind. Conditions that may occur include swallowing difficulties, peptic ulcers, gastritis, irritable bowel syndrome, and itching of the anal region. Of course, there are other factors which also contribute to these problems such as diet, infections, and poor eating habits.

Sometimes a man who is anxious often has to urinate frequently during the day. This is sometimes labeled "spastic bladder" or "irritable bladder." Typically, men suffering from this condition have to go to the bathroom repeatedly before beginning a car ride, attending an art performance, or in any situation during which emptying the bladder would be inconvenient.

Anxiety can also be expressed as worry. The andropausal male is apt to worry more than he formerly did. The list of things he worries about may seem endless. He may worry about his finances, his marriage, the welfare of his children, or problems at work. He may even, among his other worries, become obsessively concerned about his own health. He may dwell on thoughts of his own frailty and death. Every change he sees in his body may seem to him to be yet another sign of the irreversible physical decline into which he feels himself sliding. Such an awareness of physical aging is not limited to men suffering from viropause, but in them the feeling is likely to be so strong that they sometimes become obsessed with it.

Mentally healthy people will see a physician when they have concerns about their physical health. The viropausal/andropausal man, on the other hand, tends to do nothing, or delays the medical evaluation as long as possible. He is afraid that a disabling or fatal condition is progressing somewhere in his body. This idea is so unacceptable that he does nothing about it which only makes the situation worse if he is ill.

At the age when male menopause frequently has its onset, men naturally begin to think more about their own future and the future of their families. That is, of course, normal and healthy. However, to be obsessed by the worry and yet be unable to take any practical action in planning for the future is not normal. Men who are suffering from male menopause are often anxious and driven to worry but are unable to make realistic plans that will ease those worries.

Planning means making adjustments to reality and to the changes that will almost certainly come with age. Yet the anxiety that so often characterizes male menopause may impair a man's ability to think clearly. He often has unusual difficulty making decisions, and the decisions he makes may not be wise ones. If he recognizes that he is having trouble thinking clearly, that recognition can add to his anxiety. A vicious cycle can result. He may worry about not being able to think as clearly as he could formerly, and that worry can further impair his ability to think. It can be a downward spiral he can't escape from. In such cases, the problem is not organic or physical, but emotional. It is the result of anxiety or depression.

Fearfulness

Fear is a normal and often useful reaction. In threatening circumstances, it reminds us to remove ourselves from danger as part of the "flight or fight" phenomenon. Because cavemen feared the saber-tooth tiger, they ran when they saw one, thus saving their lives. Today, we exercise caution while driving our cars to avoid feared injury. However, there are some fears that arise out of psychological causes that serve little or no purpose. If we don't recognize the source of fear and do whatever is necessary to remove or get away from the cause, the fear becomes destructive.

When we arrive at middle age, thoughts of our own death may begin to creep furtively into our minds. Eventually, these thoughts may begin to occur more and more frequently and with greater intensity. If they persist, become obsessive, and produce depression, they can become a part of the viropause/andropause syndrome. Fear of aging and illness can be overwhelming for some men and can contribute to the male menopause syndrome.

One of my patients clearly showed signs of this fear. At the suggestion of his older brother, Walter Levin, age fifty-two, reluctantly arrived at my office requesting tests to rule out cancer. After his father had died of colon carcinoma a few months earlier, the entire family had been told that, in some instances, bowel cancer runs in the family.

As we talked I learned that Walter hadn't had a physical exam since he was discharged from the Marine Corps at the age of twenty-six. He had always considered himself a healthy man. He took pride in his well-proportioned, strong body. Minor illnesses were annoying because they detracted from his self-image. His pattern was to try to ignore the symptoms. He even teased his wife for "running to the doctor with every little cold."

The death of his father was unsettling because Walter had always pictured his father as a robust man. Discovering him susceptible to a devastating illness increased the already bad feelings Walter was suffering in his grieving. But even though the grief eventually decreased, his ill feelings and discontent increased. He started worrying obsessively about whether he had cancer or some other bodily defect.

Fortunately, Walter's tests were negative, but I took the opportunity to talk to him about the value of regular visits for preventing death from conditions that might be detected early and corrected. On his last visit, I felt satisfied when he indicated that he intended to come in regularly for a health evaluation.

No one likes illness, not even a doctor, and, of course, thoughts of impaired health are disturbing. In our culture, we subconsciously identify old age with a number of negative ideas, especially with declining health. In fact, we tend to picture old age as an illness instead of regarding it as a culminating stage in life. If thoughts of illness are obsessive and disproportionate to reality, they become pathological. In a man who is middle-aged, they contribute to menopausal symptoms.

When fear creates excessive worry and anxiety, it can be considered abnormal. The man experiencing male menopause may have one predominant fear that dominates him or, more commonly, a combination of meaningless fears like fears of illness, dying, reduced social status, losing respect, or losing control of life.

Non-viropausal men acknowledge these fears, seek the underlying causes, and take appropriate measures to eliminate them. Adjustment may include making changes in lifestyle, or mental adjustments such as rationalization or modifying the way the person thinks about things. During male menopause, a man may not acknowledge the presence of fears or recognize their source. Because of other mental or emotional disturbances, he may not be able to make appropriate decisions or adjustments.

When the problem of fear goes unsolved, anxiety begins or intensifies. Dysphoria may result or get worse leading to irritability, irrational behavior, self-depreciation, and other reactions further discussed in Chapter 5.

Inadequacy

Men in their forties and fifties are forced to become more realistic as society's expectations of them increase. This "reality check" often leads to negative reminders that they haven't reached all the goals they have set for themselves, that there are limitations to the heights they will achieve in life. A man's response to this realization of limits is often one of inadequacy—and if the feeling is intense or long lived, may push the man into the viropause/andropause syndrome.

A major part of male menopause is a sense of personal inadequacy. Declining sexuality and physical stamina also promote feelings of inadequacy. Understandably, the man who experiences a sudden loss of self-esteem will try to eliminate this unpleasant feeling that often leads to anxiety and/or dysphoria. The viropausal man seems to undergo a personality change, becoming irritable, cranky, and short-tempered. His daily activity pattern may change: he may sleep more, eat more and more often, drink more, shirk work responsibilities, become withdrawn, change or discontinue hobbies, and become more physically reckless or more inactive.

Some men choose to fight their feelings of inadequacy by trying to reverse what they perceive as the cause of their bad feelings. The viropausal man may decide to acquire a more youthful wardrobe or adult toys like hot tubs or expensive power tools.

It's also not surprising that men in viropause/andropause often purchase cars that provide more than just transportation. A sporty or powerful car often is bought to relieve feelings of inadequacy or failure. The purchase of a car often coincides with a new obsession about automobiles. This is demonstrated by subscribing to and reading numerous automobile magazines and books. Viropausal men may develop a preference for films with sports cars featured or car chase scenes. They might join a sports car club and participate in car rallies or races. An unrelenting compulsion to "trade up" may be overwhelming.

This same category of response may be directed to speed boats or yachts or motorcycles, or signing up for flying lessons and buying a plane. These interests all reflect the renewal of thrill by seeking the open road or the sea or the sky.

As men experiencing male menopause change their behavior patterns, they may start frequenting places where younger people congregate such as trendy bars, restaurants and travel sites. (Foreign resorts capitalize on this by installing discos, promoting nude beaches, and so on.) They may seek new friends who they believe to be of higher status—especially among the younger set.

Due to their feelings of inadequacy, ambition increases and men experiencing the viropause syndrome try hard to move higher up the work ladder. They will almost sell their souls to get a key to the executive washroom or to get on the Board of Directors while desperately identifying with their superiors or perceived superiors.

Desperation impairs the judgment of andropausal men, and they start making bad decisions, often of a financial nature. They abandon good rules of stock trading, looking to make a killing in the market or getting involved in shaky deals that eventually turn sour.

The man with symptoms of viropause may become preoccupied with his health as well as his physical appearance. Often he engages in new physical activities, especially in sports where younger people predominate, such as skiing or jogging.

Inadequacy-caused behavioral changes of the andropausal male have always provided grist for fiction and films. Our laughter at the absurd situations stems from our own experiences or from the misbehavior of spouses or friends. We may not have had a name for this behavior, but we certainly all recognize it.

Even when symptoms are not dramatic enough or severe enough to cause men to seek help from a doctor or a counselor, it is important to realize that they are possible indications of male menopause. They are signs of a specific condition that responds to treatment. For many men, a significant part of the treatment is simply getting them to see that other men have experienced similar difficulties, recovered, and gone on to live satisfying and happy lives.

For the majority of men, the middle years are a period of stress and adjustment, and often a time of crisis. There are some men for whom the stress and anxiety of mid-life are particularly acute. These men need professional help if they are to recover. For a few, male menopause becomes a chronic condition, and their anxiety and depression are persistent. The succeeding chapters will continue to demystify the viropause/andropause syndrome and will provide guidance to help make it understandable and acceptable. With acceptance comes recovery.

CHAPTER 3

Mid-Life Changes in Sexuality in the Physically Healthy Man

A man's sexuality changes during his middle years. When he becomes aware of these changes he also often begins to wonder about his future sexual life. In a society that equates sexual prowess with masculinity, that wonder can change to worry. Most men observe these changes and are not excessively troubled by them. However, for some men the worry increases and turns into fear. "Am I physically abnormal?" "Will I be able to enjoy a full sex life when I'm older?" "How is my wife going to respond to these changes?" The list of questions is endless. Sexual changes and emotional responses to those changes are a prominent part of male menopause.

Men tend to notice the physical changes in their sexuality first and the psychological changes, such as libido reduction, later on. The most common changes in sexuality that occur in the forties and fifties are failure to have an erection in circumstances that previously were associated with erection, less firmness of the penis during an erection, occasional loss of erection during sexual activity, delayed orgasm, failure to achieve an orgasm, reduced force of ejaculation, and reduced volume of ejaculate.

Feelings of sexual inadequacy are a common component of the viropause/andropause syndrome. At the first sign of even slight sexual decline, the concern begins. It may be an insignificant reduction in libido, a single erection failure, or a slight weakening in orgasmic power. These concerns grow until they produce a sense of inadequacy.

Stimulation

During the early teenage years, a boy develops considerable sexuality. Libido increases rapidly. Thoughts of sex pop into his mind many times during the day. He has erections with little or no physical stimulation of the penis. It takes very little auditory or visual stimulation to start an erection.

But for the older man, erection response is likely to require considerably more stimulation. Frequently, both physical stimulus of the penis and other sensory input are necessary. Such stimulation may be visual, auditory, or tactile, such as the feel of a female body against his. When a middle-aged man notices that his erection is not immediate and that he requires increased stimulation, it may become a cause of concern.

When a man understands that this need for additional stimulation is not a negative change and that all forms of stimulation provide an additional degree of pleasure and the pleasure is prolonged, his fears subside. There is more kissing, hugging, caressing, fondling, and stroking. There is more verbal expression of love and "sex talk." Thus the act of intercourse is more fun and exciting. As a man becomes aware of these new pleasures, he embraces the newly discovered benefits of the changes. (Most younger men can hardly wait to "get it in" and in their hurry are not good lovers, missing much of the pleasure of extended sexual activity.)

However, without this knowledge the viropausal man views the changes as evidence of aging and loss of masculinity and becomes convinced that complete sexual failure is near. He needs to know that, though it may take more stimulation than it once did, these are normal changes and that the typical man is able for many years—sometimes as long as he lives— to develop an erection.

Erection

In many cultures, a large, very hard penis has been identified with masculinity and sexual satisfaction. However, most of us know that it is merely a cultural myth. In mid-life, however, the degree of firmness of the erection may decrease slightly, and this may be distressing to the man who believes this change is progressive. In the normal male between forty and sixty, a decrease in firmness in the range of five to twenty percent is common; but unless this is a disease such as diabetes present, it rarely goes as high as even a fifty percent decrease—and there is never a hundred percent decrease. The degree of decrease at mid-life depends on a variety of factors such as mental fatigue, distractions, duration and intensity of foreplay, physical surroundings, and the consumption of drugs or alcohol. Fortunately, erections remain adequate for insertion and thrusting throughout the life of the normal male.

A young man can develop a full erection in a few seconds whereas it may take several minutes, sometimes as long as a half hour, for an older man to do so. The younger man never loses an erection except when he is distracted (for example, when someone walks into the room during masturbation). In later life a man may occasionally "lose it" during intercourse. There are various reasons for this. Some distractions can reverse an erection: the phone ringing, a door slamming nearby, furtive thoughts of other responsibilities or unfinished work, or even distracting words from a partner.

Loss of the erection can be especially distressing to the middle-aged man because the urge to continue coitus remains in spite of "going soft" and because a man may also be concerned about his inability to satisfy his partner. Loss of erection during intercourse does occur occasionally but is seldom a frequent problem for a healthy man. It presents no major problems for a happy, well-adjusted couple once they are informed and realize this may normally occur now and then. It is reassuring to know that this is not a harbinger of further sexual impairment.

A forty-seven-year-old patient of mine, Ted Daniels, expressed concern to me about his sexuality during a routine physical examination. Several times over the past six months he had not been able to get an erection even though he greatly wanted intercourse with his wife. He offered additional history in response to my questions:

Ted's first erectile failure had occured five years previously when he had drunk too much, and others had happened three or four more times in the following years. When failure occured several times in six months, it began to worry him. He began obsessing about it when he and his wife watched a movie that included sensual scenes. It nagged at him when he and his wife were preparing for bed. "I'm almost afraid to go to bed, knowing there might be sex."

Ted's history demonstrates what I as a physician have found to be the most common cause of impotence: fear of failure. Any kind of fear suppresses libido and, with each failure, fear is intensified. If I had not asked about his sex life, Ted's fear and related failures might have gone on for years with disastrous consequences.

I asked some more questions about the circumstances surrounding the first failures. Ted told me most of them occured at bedtime at the end of a particularly stressful work day. When I asked about his intake of alcohol, he said he often had an extra shot of liquor after an especially hard day. But when asked about his sexual performance on holidays, he brightened and told me that two weeks earlier he and his wife had "great sex, as good as ever" while on a long weekend at a nearby resort.

My examination of Ted and the lab tests showed no physical cause for Ted's erectile failure. I tried to reassure him and gave him some material on the subject to read at home. When he returned for a follow-up visit, we discussed normal sexual maturation and what could be expected over subsequent decades. I gave him some advice regarding alcohol consumption, stress, and good health practices as they relate to libido and sexual performance. I encouraged him to share the information and his thoughts with his wife.

Orgasm and Ejaculation

In his early sexual life, a man is almost always able to experience a climax. Older men occasionally may not have an orgasm for no apparent reason. Occasionally there are some underlying causes. The most common factors are fatigue and fear of not reaching a satisfactory termination of the sexual act. But once two partners become informed and realize this is a normal event for a healthy aging male, they can readily accept it.

A young man may be able to ejaculate a large amount of semen with considerable force. The amount depends on how much time has elapsed since the previous ejaculation. The organs producing the fluids work at a fairly steady rate, so if the previous ejaculation is recent the amount will be less. The older man produces seminal fluid at a slower rate so the volume is decreased. In addition, the involuntary muscles used in ejaculation may not be as strong in the older man, so the force may be lessened. These changes do not decrease the sensation or satisfaction experienced during orgasm. There is no problem unless a man notes this change in quantity and force of ejaculation and believes the changes are evidence of decreasing masculinity and fears it may be progressive. At times, older men do not have the strong compelling urge for orgasm that characterizes the sexual act of the younger male. The feeling of frustration is not as strong.

The reasons for the decrease in orgasmic urge as a man grows older are not well understood. The causes may be partly physical, such as less physical pressure on the organs of ejaculation. More likely, the cause is psychological. However, as a man realizes that ejaculation does not reflect on his masculinity, he will be less troubled by not having an orgasm. When feelings of love and affection are strong, they are not diminished by the absence of ejaculation.

Diverging Sexuality

In the early teen years a man's sexual activity is usually confined to masturbation. There is sexual daydreaming and interest in explicit pictures, movies, and so on. As the male grows older, his spectrum of sexual activity enlarges. Today, by the late teen years, most males have engaged in intercourse and have experimented with various modes of sexual stimulation.

In their twenties, most men make considerable effort to achieve sexual gratification. This may include working to acquire the accessories believed necessary to this end, such as an attractive automobile and fashionable clothes. Men may select and marry a woman partially because of their conscious or unconscious sexual drive. They may also study and practice skills to become "good lovers."

At about age thirty, a man's sexuality reaches its greatest height. It then wanes slightly for the next ten years and then decreases rapidly for the next twenty. There are many explanations for this precipitous decrease, but an important one is the intervening and disrupting concerns with achieving financial stability, as well as the desire to improve status in the family, community, and society in general. This leaves men less time and energy for sex.

At the end of this period of a man's life (forty to sixty), sexuality gradually declines. Increased awareness of other changes of age worsens the viropause/andropause syndrome. Often a wife who is forty to fifty is experiencing increased sexuality while her husband's sexual desire is decreasing. This divergence frequently becomes apparent to the husband. As a result, he may develop feelings of frustration and inadequacy. This can be a real source of anxiety.

CHAPTER 3

If unrecognized and not appropriately dealt with, this difference between the husband's and wife's desires for sex often becomes a source of marital conflict. To avoid or remove the conflict, a couple must communicate their feelings. The couple must admit there is a divergence in sexuality, talk about it, and seek ways to handle it. Both should be willing to make some adjustments and concessions to handle the change. For instance, a wife may occasionally suppress her sexual desire and a husband may occasionally perform sex even when he is not in the mood.

Another kind of sexuality divergence came to my attention when Harry Wilson, fifty-seven, came to my office. He was a year overdue for his annual physical examination. His wife, Pam, used this as an excuse to get him in to see me. During her annual gynecological exam I asked a routine question: "Do you have pelvic pain with intercourse?" She hesitated before answering, then said, "I hardly know how to answer that; we haven't done it for over a year."

Pam went on to explain that her husband didn't seem interested anymore, but that she still had sexual urges which she relieved with masturbation. She felt no guilt using this means of sexual release, but was saddened that she and Harry no longer expressed their love in bed. He was a loving, caring husband but "just didn't seem to need it anymore." She admitted she had not shared her thoughts with him because she didn't want to hurt his feelings.

Their differing needs and desires for sex were a common mid-life problem. When I recommended that some counseling could re-establish a healthy sexual relationship, she asked how to go about it. I suggested a good starting point would be a physical examination for Harry and at that time I would take a sex history.

During Harry's general health evaluation he gave a fairly common history of sexual abstinence for a man in his late fifties. His first comment was "I suppose a man of my age should not expect to need sex," but he hastened to add that his interest in sex had not disappeared.

About the time his two children went off to college, Pam developed "female problems." She had had abnormal intermittent vaginal bleeding for over a year. A hysterectomy eliminated these symptoms, but the entire episode of pain, bleeding, and surgery left Harry apprehensive about his wife's health and her sexual organs.

During the sixteen months of his wife's illness and surgery, Harry chose not to make sexual advances. He didn't consider this a sacrifice as his sexual drives were not normally high and were sublimated by caring for her and demonstrating his affection in non-physical ways. I asked him how he felt about his wife now that the surgery was over and she had fully recovered. "Do you feel that intercourse might hurt her or damage her? Do you feel she is less feminine? Do you feel less physically attracted to her?" His answers were vague; apparently he had not considered these aspects. I got the impression he had subconsciously avoided thinking about them.

Harry's tests provided no evidence of a physical explanation for his low level of sexual desire. When I asked him, "Would you be interested in re-establishing sexual relations with your wife?" he responded with a very definite yes. I scheduled an appointment for the couple to come in together so we could talk about their sexual history and consider counseling. I reassured them there would be no unfavorable effects on her pelvis if they resumed intercourse.

Ten days later, Harry called me and said they had

decided against seeing a counselor because they were having intercourse and "it was wonderful; better than ever before."

When Pam's pelvic problems started, Harry had begun thinking of his wife as a frail person and started treating her accordingly. In this case, I suspect that his wife's increasing sexuality was a significant factor in solving the problems of a sexually dysfunctional relationship.

Libido

Male patterns of libido change when they are in their forties and fifties. During this period of life, external forces are changing—forces that affect sexual appetite. When competing forces are small libido increases, but when competing forces are greater, libido decreases. Other interests often include a man's occupation, but personal interests also come into play. If life at home takes on a routine pattern without much variation, libido may decrease. Introduction of a new sexual interest, sexual variation, or a new partner will increase libido.

Even when there are no significant external influences, a man's libido goes through a gradual decrease during his forties and fifties. I estimate the decrease to be about five percent for each five-year increment. That is, the appetite for sex in the average healthy male will decrease by twenty percent between the ages of forty and sixty. The rate of decrease decelerates after sixty. If there is an outlet for stimulating sexual release, libido decreases very little in the "golden years."

A man's baseline libido, established in his twenties, is usually the controlling factor of his lifetime sexual desire. The man who has intercourse daily at twenty-five will probably want it three or four times a week when he is fifty-five. On the other hand, the man who has intercourse once a week at twenty-five may only want it once every two weeks in his fifties.

However, significant changes in libido can be physical in origin.

At his annual examination, Dick Millburn, a forty-seven-year-old longtime patient of mine, and I exchanged pleasantries. However, I noticed that under the banter his mood was unhappy and he seemed nervous. His age and profile suggested male menopause. I began asking my usual questions about his health: "Are you functioning satisfactorily sexually?" "Are you having erections and orgasms?" "Is there any decrease in libido?" Fidgeting in his chair, Dick looked away and said softly, "Glad you asked. I must be getting old. My need for sex has almost disappeared."

Dick had had an insurance examination eighteen months earlier that indicated high blood pressure. When he came to me at that time I performed the usual medical workup and determined he had essential hypertension. His blood pressure responded very nicely to medication and improved health habits.

When he reported sexual dysfunction, I strongly suspected it was due to hypertension medication. I discussed my theory with Dick and told him that hypertension medication and excessive alcohol consumption are the most common drug-induced causes of sexual impairment. I also explained that many effective blood-pressure-lowering medications are now available, and although some may impair sexual function in some men, others may not. It sometimes requires several visits to find the best one and adjust the dosage properly.

Over the course of several more office visits we discussed his other symptoms of male menopause and stabilized his blood pressure. He happily reported that his libido had returned to its previous level.

Anxiety About Libido

Libido is defined as sexual desire: the energy derived from primitive impulses, and sexual urge or instinct. In everyday language it is often referred to as the appetite for sex, and it is similar to a person's appetite for food. After eating or sex, the appetite decreases. After a strong stimulus (for example, exposure to eroticisms) sexual appetite returns quickly in spite of satisfaction. Some people have greater cravings for food or sex than others. There can be craving for certain foods or types of sex. There are variations in appetite for food or sex for any individual during the course of the day as well as during the course of a lifetime.

Persons who experience anxiety have reduced libido. It is as though the mind is saying, "No way can I think of sex when I'm so upset." The thought processes necessary for a healthy sexual appetite are crowded out by disturbing thoughts that fill the mind of the anxious man.

Anxiety is a common disorder. People use various words and phrases when referring to their feelings that are indications they are suffering from anxiety. They may refer to themselves as being nervous, anxious, apprehensive, uptight, stressed, under tension, or shaky inside. All of us experience anxiety to some degree every day. When it occurs with real causes, that is, when it is the result of stressors, it is a normal response. When it occurs without an identifiable cause it is abnormal. In addition, when the degree of response to stressors is unreasonable, it is abnormal. There are several different types of anxiety. They include generalized anxiety, adjustment disorder anxiety, social anxiety, various phobias, panic and agoraphobia. Generalized anxiety is the type that often produces sexual dysfunction.

Almost every patient who experiences anxiety can relate his bad feelings to some problem in his life. The most common problems are related to work, personal relationships, and real (or perceived) illness. When the response to the problem is inappropriate, we physicians consider it an illness. And this illness can be destructive to normal sexual function.

Anxiety produces mental fatigue, and this type of fatigue is a strong deterrent to sexual function. Mental fatigue, with or without anxiety, is a very common cause of reduced libido and impotence. On the other hand, physical fatigue, unless extreme, does not impair sexual function.

Job problems often create barriers to satisfying sex. The man who gets a pink slip or fears that he may is naturally anxious, as is the man who develops a physical symptom without physical basis and worries that it may be evidence of a serious disease. His fear-laden thoughts create an indestructible barrier to thoughts of sex, and his libido drops. The worry produces anxiety, which reduces his libido, and he may become sexually dysfunctional. His wife, in an attempt to take his mind off his worries, may make a sexual advance which he rejects. She may then feel that he is rejecting her, not rejecting sex.

Anxiety is often treated by the use of sedatives or tranquilizers. While they relieve the feelings of anxiety, they are not appropriate in the treatment of sexual problems. It is important to know that these medications, like alcohol, may interfere with normal mental and physical activity needed for good sexual performance.

Mental Fatigue

A man whose job requires constant, high-pressure attention is mentally fatigued at the end of the day. In an effort to escape the responsibilities of the day, he may be inclined to escape by stopping at a bar after he leaves work or pouring himself a drink when he arrives home. Some workers relieve their mental fatigue by substituting the more pleasant physical fatigue of aerobic activity after work.

Unless extreme, physical fatigue is not a hindrance to sex. After hours on the slopes, the skier often feels very libidinous. Even a few beers won't diminish his sexual capabilities. On the other hand, the mentally fatigued man does not have the emotional reserves needed for sex. Because the physical changes required for erection and orgasm have their beginning in the psyche, if his psyche is depleted by mental fatigue, his sexual ability will be reduced or absent and his libido will be decreased. If the mentally fatigued man uses excessive amounts of alcohol in an attempt to relieve his fatigue, there is an additional impediment to sex.

Sexual Inadequacy

The man experiencing male menopause demonstrates a variety of responses to his supposed sexual inadequacy, but the underlying motive is to prove that he is not losing his sexuality. Responses may include going on a health kick (dieting or exercise program), which some forms of advertising promotes as a sure cure for waning sexuality. He may change his dress pattern as he looks for the ultimate complimentary item. Often, a self-forced increase in sexual activity is tried. This activity may be masturbation or sexual encounters with his wife or someone else. He may encourage his partner to participate in sexual experimentation, sometimes by introducing a drug into the encounters. Increased use of alcohol may be tried to reduce inhibitions and allow new sexual exploration. He may begin using pornographic stimulants, books, magazines, or videos.

These responses can be considered normal when used within the confines of reasonable limits and are not self-destructive or other-destructive. However, they must be considered abnormal, and evidence of andropause, when they go beyond the limits of taste or safety.

Sexual activity can occur no matter how old one is, but the intensity of sexuality changes for everyone. For normal individuals, change does not mean stagnation. Most of us benefit by a healthy sexual attitude and practice. The gradual diminution of sexuality is usually accepted and is of little concern to most people.

When a man in his forties or fifties recognizes and accepts the change in his sexual tempo, he can be reassured that there is no subsequent, precipitous slowing. He can also take comfort from the occasional stellar performance. It's reassuring to him when, on holiday, his libido seems insatiable. He is happy to find his wife responds as well when his erection is not as "big and hard" and he is relieved when she remains undisturbed by the occasional failure and still loves him. Fears are allayed and self-confidence regained when a man learns that the slight physical modifications of sexual function are universal. They do not presage the end of sexual life or diminish his masculinity.

The normal man, as he ages, experiences some changes

in sexuality, but they are slight. More stimulus is needed to have an erection. Tumescence is usually less and occasional erection failure occurs. Delayed orgasm or failure to achieve orgasm may also occur. Reduced libido or sex drive is part of the sexuality change, though it varies considerably from man to man, and from day to day for the individual. Daily anxiety and stress can temporarily reduce the libido. If this is a long-term problem, professional help is recommended.

CHAPTER 4

What Causes Andropause

Medical practitioners have always sought to discover the causes of disease. Understanding the cause is necessary to finding a cure and, more importantly, to learning how to prevent disease. For example, the discovery of bacteria and how to deal with them has substantially reduced human suffering. Diseases such as typhoid are now curable and also preventable. But research has mostly focused on physical ailments. Progress in researching the causes of psychological ills has been less spectacular.

As of 1993, the etiology has evaded those who have studied the illness. A discussion of the subject of causes is interesting, but remains speculative.

Researchers know that andropause is a significant problem among men in societies of the industrialized nations. Conversely, there are societies in which viropause/andropause is so rare that it is almost nonexistent. These, for the most part, are in the non-industrialized countries where the cultures might be thought of as primitive. The male menopause syndrome is more common where traditions and customs are weak than where they are strong. We also know that andropause is more apt to affect men who have high ambition and drive and who have had considerable success in their lives, though it is not limited to such men. Research also shows that andropause is most evident among urban populations. It is less common where people live in small communities or in villages or where there is a traditional lifestyle.

On a small Greek island I visit, Nikolas Karapoulos, fifty-six, owns and operates one of the five *tavernas* in a town of a few hundred people. His father was the previous owner of the business and continues to help his son during the busy hours. Nikolas's wife and middle son also work with him. None of them has ever lived any place other than this island.

Except for the tourists, the population is stable. The islanders' income is derived primarily from tourism, diving for sponges, and fishing. Very little has changed in the surroundings or lifestyle of the inhabitants for centuries. Nikolas and his family are happy and content. They have compatible relationships with one another and with the other members of their community, including with their competitors.

Male menopause is nonexistent among the men on this island. The transition through the various stages of life are smooth with minimal mental anguish. The men tend to have a high level of sexuality but keep it well within the confines of propriety.

Retirement is a foreign concept to these men. They work as long as they are physically able and are proud to be part of the working community. Nikolas and others like him are content to be working at the same jobs their fathers had. This isn't to say they aren't industrious. The entrepreneurial spirit is there—Nikolas works hard to get the tourist business.

Though alcohol is readily available and inexpensive, the island men tend to drink moderately and seldom get drunk; the women barely drink at all. At the Saturday night parties there is drinking, but most entertainment centers on music, dancing, and brisk conversation. The parties are attended by those of all ages. The first dancers on the floor after dinner are the children—some just old enough to walk. Later, they fall asleep on mattresses provided by their parents or in their parents' arms.

There is no dread of aging. When islanders become infirm with age, their children and other members of their community gladly care for them. The old are well respected by the younger members of the community. These are a religious people who seem to have no undue fear or negative feelings about death. The respect for elders goes beyond life as indicated by a long and intense period of mourning.

The social and cultural attitudes, as well as the healthy lifestyles, of Nikolas and his fellow townsmen may explain the absence of any discernible viropause/andropause syndrome on this Greek island.

Goals

Some studies suggest that the goal orientation of men of Western cultures and certain Eastern cultures provides an explanation for male menopause. Where the influence of these cultures is strongest, young people, especially young men, are encouraged to set high goals for themselves. They are encouraged to become financially and socially successful. They are taught to plan their lives in such a way as to secure status and economic success for themselves and their families. They are encouraged to strive toward goals that are not easily achievable. "Dream big," they are urged. "Attempt the impossible." "A man's reach should exceed his grasp."

One message in particular that young men hear is that they should strive for a higher status than their fathers achieved. If they don't, their lack of ambition may be considered a failure. The factory worker's son hopes to own the factory someday. He is not expected to be satisfied with simply being as good a worker as his father was.

At forty-four, Emil Morris was the assistant sales manager for a small business when he came to my office complaining of headaches. A physical examination and laboratory tests revealed no significant abnormality, so I concluded the headaches were due to tight muscles in the head and neck (muscle contraction headache).

Because these headaches are occasionally psychosomatic, I took additional history. For several months Emil had frequently been awakening at two or three in the morning and then not being able to return to sleep. His wife had begun complaining of his increasing irritability. Emil was easygoing by nature, but his wife now noted he had a "short fuse." He himself had become aware of getting upset easily in response to minor annoyances.

Nine months previously, Emil had been overlooked for a promotion to sales manager. A new man was brought in and given the job. Emil was reluctant to admit it, but he still felt considerable resentment.

After two counseling visits during which we talked at length about his feelings, Emil recognized his lingering resentment as the cause of his anxiety. After two additional sessions, he acknowledged that there was a deeper reason for the resentment: It had become apparent to him that he was not going to enjoy the business success he had hoped for when he joined the firm.

As Emil did, the man experiencing andropause develops anxiety with lesser cause than a normal man and it tends to be more serious and last longer. Minor disappointments and setbacks in the lives of healthy men cause only slight and short-lived periods of anxiety. Andropausal men do not respond to the usual anxiety reducers: vacations, encouragement from family and friends, rationalizations, and priority adjustments. The longer the anxiety endures, the more importance he assigns to its apparent cause and the insult he perceives to his well-being. Physical symptoms frequently become an added annoyance.

After Emil had verbalized his thoughts, he better understood his feelings and became more realistic about his potential for advancement. Five months later, when he came to my office about a minor skin condition, he volunteered, "Life has smoothed out." The headaches were now infrequent.

Setting high goals cannot be regarded as altogether bad. It is, in fact, necessary for greatness, whether in an individual or a nation. However, it isn't always possible to achieve our dreams. In fact, most of us don't. And there comes a time, usually in mid-life, when a man who looks at himself and his achievements realizes that he cannot reach the degree of success that he had hoped for. He may find himself standing at some lower peak of a mountain he had started to climb and have to admit that he can't make it to the summit—that time is running out. There is a feeling of frustration and disappointment when he compares himself to other men, or when he compares his achievements to his original goals. The disappointment can be devastating. This disillusionment can negatively affect his emotional adjustment to middle age.

The greater the difference between actual achievement and a man's original goals, the greater the devastation. The schedules men set for themselves to realize their goals can vary by decades, so their self-evaluated failure can occur early or late in mid-life. This schedule variation may be one explanation for the similar disparity in the age of the onset of viropause.

Studies also suggest that the consumer-oriented world we have built for ourselves contributes to this male syndrome. Materialism has its effect. Advertising and marketing have become integral to our lives, part and parcel of our values. We are consumers as well as producers and our identities become connected to what we want to consume. Media messages shape the forms our desires take. We are tempted, aggressively and continuously it seems, by all kinds of hype. We want more than we can possibly have, and we even want what we should not have. We are seduced into believing that we should have more than we truly need.

In her book *Are They Selling Her Lips*, clinical psychologist Dr. Carol Moog discusses the excesses of today's advertising. Moog illustrates how advertisers manipulate consumers by developing an overwhelming feeling of need for their products.

Consider, for instance, the advertising for automobiles. The choices of vehicles we can buy include cars, trucks, motorcycles, and motor homes. The actual reasons to choose a particular vehicle include comfort, cost, efficiency, reliability, and lifestyle. But these are seldom what advertisers use to motivate purchases. Advertising tries to make us believe that we need—indeed, must have—a particular car, not because it is economical or reliable, but because it is "us," because it fills an emotional need we have to see ourselves as a certain kind of person. This projected image of a car owner often includes an implied promise of increased sexuality. Those who are insecure about their status are most susceptible to sales promotions based on emotional needs rather than on real needs; and the susceptible include men in their middle years who are concerned about their self-image, achievements, and masculinity.

When men in viropause are surrounded by such advertising, virtually immersed in it, their feelings of dissatisfaction and of unmet needs are likely to grow. The craving for more than they have can lead to frustration. It can make them more dissatisfied with who they are and what they have achieved. Male menopause may be, in part, a result of the unrealistic expectations that modern merchandising encourages when it teaches us to be forever dissatisfied. The man experiencing viropause is especially susceptible to the hype. With repeated exposure to such advertising the feeling of need grows. The craving for more can lead to extravagance, which in turn can promote financial problems. Advertising also encourages a lifestyle that is damaging to our health; for example, using tobacco, overeating, and drinking too much. Advertising, obviously, has a strong influence on all of us, especially the young and immature, when setting goals. It contributes to high expectations and unrealistic lifestyles that can crash back on men in their middle years in the form of andropause.

Aging

If a man's discovery that he can't realize his ambitions coincides with his discovery that his body isn't as reliable and as strong as it once was, the effects of male menopause are compounded. An awareness of the irreversibility of aging can surprise a man who has always prided himself on his fitness and strength.

While we are young we become aware of our bodies' appearance and vigor. A self-image is created. During early life, the body recovers rapidly and completely from injury and illness. We acknowledge this phenomenon subconsciously. (Maybe this, at least partially, explains the reckless behavior of some youths.) As we grow older our bodies recover and heal more slowly. Eventually, the time comes when an illness becomes chronic or an injury results in a permanent, inconvenient disability. Acknowledging such irreversible physical change can be especially devastating when some pleasure of life must be given up—certain sports, some foods, unlimited travel, or hobbies, for example.

Men dislike the appearance of aging in their faces and bodies. Being forced to recognize physical changes can be devastating to the ego. In our society, doing something about deteriorating appearance is acceptable for women. It is less acceptable for men. Some women tint their hair, have cosmetic surgery, wear support undergarments, and so on to camouflage the changes of aging. These changes are usually accepted by family, friends, and community. These same changes are less acceptable for the aging male. (Interestingly, when young men change the color and style of their hair, their peers see it as "cool.")

One of my patients had a particularly difficult time

accepting the changes of aging. Larry McIntyre, a fifty-six-year-old producer of television films, came to my office for treatment of sunburn. He had signed up for a series of twice weekly sessions at the local tanning salon in preparation for a trip he and his wife were planning to the Mexican Riviera. A graduated program of exposure was outlined for him, but he became impatient because he didn't think he was getting the desired deep tan fast enough. The salon wisely limited the duration of ultraviolet exposure, so he went to a second salon for additional sessions. He had received a double dose of ultraviolet the day before his visit to my office and had developed an uncomfortable sunburn over most of his body.

When I walked into the examination room, I immediately noticed a big difference in Larry's appearance since the last time I had seen him. His head was covered with many small curls. As long as I had known him, Larry had had straight hair combed in a traditional style. He was aware of my interest and explained he liked his wife's new perm so he got one, too. After this visit, I wondered if Larry was entering viropause, but he seemed happy and excited about his planned trip, so I dismissed it from my mind.

The last week he was in Mexico, Larry's trip was spoiled by an episode of diarrhea. Some annoying abdominal cramps persisted into his second week back home which he consulted me about. While I was examining him, he proudly showed me a new heavy gold chain and medallion that he had bought in Mexico at a "great bargain price of only $1,400."

During this visit, I noticed that the exuberance that Larry had shown during his last visit had faded and he appeared dejected. I asked him about his trip. "Oh, it was okay, but it was boring after the first few days. To make things worse, my wife wanted to take side trips, and when I said I didn't want to, she got angry and unloaded on me. She told me that I hadn't been any fun for months."

I asked him if he thought it was true that he was no fun. He confessed he had been feeling down and was worrying too much. I then asked if he wanted to schedule another appointment to talk about it and he seemed relieved that I was willing to discuss his depressed mood.

During our next visit together, I asked Larry whether he felt any differently lately. Typical of the man entering male menopause, Larry was slow to acknowledge that there had been a change. Only after four months of counseling was he able to accept the fact that he had become moody and depressed. He went through the usual reactions of denial and resentment. At that point he concluded that he was moody in response to some aging changes and vehemently announced, "I'm not going to let myself get old."

After several visits I began to discuss andropause with him. I talked about the causes, and he began to see how he fit into the pattern. Somewhat reluctantly he admitted that some of his behavior "probably was abnormal." He took some printed information on andropause home with him. On his last counseling visit he told me he had his "act together" and could see recovery in the near future.

To those men such as Larry who place a high value on their appearance, confronting the changes that aging produces is disturbing. The higher the value of appearance, the greater the disturbance. Some of the changes that bring distress are balding and gray hair, skin wrinkles, spotting of the skin on the face and hands, dental deterioration, lost skin tone and muscle tone, and the shifting of normal fat deposits from extremities to the abdomen.

There is a typical sequence of thought patterns in response to a man's first awareness of aging. First there is rejection: "There's some mistake; this really isn't happening to me." Then anger: "I'm too young for this. I don't deserve this. It's not fair. I'm going to fight it all the way." Then acceptance: "I guess I really have reached *that* age. I will have to slow down. I can have a good and happy life even though I'm slowing down and I haven't reached all of my goals." Finally comes adjustment, which includes a more realistic assessment of priorities and values. The love of family and an increased appreciation of the world around us becomes important. Part of this adjustment is acknowledging that life does eventually "run out" but that there are many good and contented years left. It makes sense to retard aging changes as much as possible, but it also makes sense to accept the limitations imposed by changes in the body and mind.

Seeing the irreversible changes of aging, the andropausal male is thrown into a state of despair. Men who are not affected by the male climacteric see these changes, accept them, and do not suffer.

Andropausal symptoms usually begin during the rejection and anger phases of this sequence. Though there is no solid evidence to prove aging is a causative factor in male menopause, it makes good sense to explore the connection.

Hormonal Changes and Impotence

Between the ages of forty-eight and seventy, men can expect a thirty to forty percent reduction in hormones, testosterone, and dihydrotestosterone, a substance produced by the metabolism of testosterone. Because the diminution in male sex hormones occurs later in life, it is rarely a factor in andropause. For men in their geriatric years, this hormonal loss can affect their bone metabolism (similar to the effect the loss of estrogen has on post-menopausal women). Men may become more susceptible to osteoporosis, which puts them at greater risk for bone fractures. Other tissues, such as muscles, can also deteriorate. Post-andropausal men may also become more subdued as their normal male aggressiveness, which is promoted by their male hormones, is reduced. The important point here is that andropause, a primarily psychological condition, occurs before the testosterone reductions do.

The two most common endocrine (hormonal) factors in order of impotence are testosterone deficiency and hyperpolactactinemia syndrome, a condition in which there is an excess of pituitary hormone which inhibits the output of testosterone. However, these hormonal abnormalities cause impotence in probably only two to five percent of cases in otherwise healthy andropausal men between ages forty and sixty. This percentage does rise significantly when there is chronic disease or deleterious habits. Diagnosis is easily established with blood tests, and both conditions respond satisfactorily to medications.

Impotence is a common factor in andropause, but hormonal deficiency rarely explains it. In the November 1991 issue of *Scientific American*, Dr. Daniel D. Federman states, "Psychogenic [mental] factors are thought to be the most frequent cause of impotence."

The results of some recent studies concerning testosterone deficiency as it relates to impotence have received wide and sensational attention in the news media. The implication in these stories has been that a reduced testicular production of testosterone is the cause of more than half the cases of impotence. However, most clinicians continue to assert that a low testosterone level causes only a small percentage of cases of impotency.

The recent studies that have been reported were mostly conducted on older men who were beyond the andropausal age. Beyond sixty, the level of testosterone in otherwise healthy men gradually declines. For some of these men, administration of testosterone will restore potency. (Additional physiological and psychological effects of testosterone are discussed in Chapter 10.)

Testosterone has a potent effect on the mind. The increase in libido in both men and women is primarily due to the mental effects of testosterone. However, the extent of the mental aspects of testosterone and how those aspects influence a man's potency have not been fully researched. There is general agreement in the scientific world that orgasms are psychologically mediated. It is men's thoughts, not physical stimulation, that triggers the process of ejaculation. The nerves in the penis send tactile messages via the spinal cord to the brain about the pleasurable sensations they're feeling. The brain responds with a message to the pelvic organs to the effect of "This feels good; go for it; ejaculate!"

Thoughts and memories contribute to the directive to ejaculate. The brain processes many complex inputs about love, affection, past experiences, and other sensory data, in addition to the message from the penis, and channels all of them into the nerve order to ejaculate. If there are impediments to the thought process, orgasm may not occur.

When a man is experiencing male menopause, he often has one or more negative thoughts that can crowd out those needed to produce an orgasm. The most common initiating event of andropause is a decrease, or perceived decrease, in sexual function. Even the slightest decline in sexuality can trigger a series of negative thoughts about inadequacies, fear of impairment of other bodily functions, and concerns about unattained goals.

When a man becomes aware of his reduced sexuality, it is usually with a great sense of loss. For some men, that loss is devastating. All men are acutely aware of their sexuality from childhood on. It is an important part of their self-image. This natural awareness is nurtured further by societal pressures. Some men are able to accept their sexuality changes and make appropriate adjustments in their lifestyles and priorities. Those who don't adjust are often pitched into the viropause/andropause syndrome.

Reduced sexuality can take a variety of forms:

1. Less awareness of visual, olfactory, and tactile sexual stimuli—the sexy appearance of women, pornographic pictures, perfumes, the pleasant odors generated by the female body, the touch of female body parts.

2. Less responsiveness—more or stronger stimuli needed to produce sexual thoughts, arouse and maintain an erection, experience orgasm, repeat the sexual act, appreciate the relaxation following climax.

3. Less verbal enjoyment—conversations that have sexual connotations, talking about sexual matters with a lover.

4. Less sexual projection—sexual body language, clothing that invites a sexual response from women.

The effect of real or perceived sexual inadequacies and

impotence on the viropausal/andropausal man cannot be overstressed. Sexual inadequacy and the psyche of the andropausal man interact in many significant ways. Reduced sexuality can cause or worsen the menopausal condition while andropause can precipitate or increase the severity of sexual inadequacy. The interaction of the two create a self-perpetuating downward spiral.

Retirement

Some aspects of retirement can contribute to the onset of male menopause. At some time during their forties or fifties, men begin to think about retirement and most start making logical and useful plans. Retirement is usually anticipated as a wonderful event in their lives. However, fear and misgiving of the retirement years ahead may be an uncomfortable response for some.

Some of the negative features of retirement years fill the mind of the man experiencing male menopause. If his work has been pleasurable and rewarding, he may look at retirement as a frightening change. This especially is true if he has not established other enjoyable occupations or hobbies by this time. The idea of becoming a second-class citizen is very distasteful. These uncomfortable thoughts are worsened by observing an unsuccessful retirement in a parent or older friend. He may unhappily dwell on this, whereas the non-andropausal male will feel joy in seeing the happiness and usefulness of other older males.

Fears

It's easy to speculate on societal circumstances and the effects they have on us in later life. In a society where there is much emphasis on the joys of youth, one can expect those in the aging segment of the population to develop feelings of inferiority. Advertising encourages us to equate happiness with youth. Even in the advertising directed at retired consumers, the more youthful-appearing geriatric folks are portrayed. We are led to believe only the young are truly happy and as one ages, happiness and joy give way to, at best, contentment and peace.

In many more developed societies there is a lower regard for older members. In some of the less developed countries the senior members of a family and society are respected and honored more than are the seniors in other countries. Even within one country differences are easily seen. In rural areas, older people are usually treated with more respect than in metropolitan areas. In a country that becomes industrialized rapidly, the status levels of the elderly change. We are seeing this shift in Japan. In the United States a high value is placed on an individual's physical appearance, and aging changes are not easily accepted. Thus American men have a harder time adjusting to the deterioration of their bodies.

A relatively new fear has joined the possible causes of andropause. In the last two decades more wives have entered the job market, and many are very successful. In some marriages, the wife's career success also has the effect of displacing the husband's conventionally dominant role in the home. When men in their forties and fifties see this happening to themselves, their friends, and colleagues, it causes apprehension about their marriages and undermines self-confidence.

Frank Latimer, who was forty-seven, was a new patient when he came to my office with multiple physical symptoms. His chief concern was "just not feeling up to par." The physical symptoms were mild and his description of them was vague. He was afraid that he had some serious generalized disease like diabetes. The results of his examination and laboratory tests were all negative.

Ten months previously, Frank had moved to my community from a neighboring state. His wife had been teaching in a community college when she was offered a higher paying position in the local college. The new job represented a big advancement in the academic world. Frank and his wife agreed that it was an offer they couldn't let pass. Frank had held a managerial job in a construction company and had been confident of finding work in the new location. However, the demand for men with his training and experience was very limited locally. He became discouraged after five months of interviewing, so he went back to his old job and commuted weekends to be with his wife.

On this commuter regimen, Frank's sleep pattern was altered. He was not eating a balanced diet, he neglected his exercise program, and he began drinking more. He developed indigestion, headaches, listlessness, and fatigue. He and his wife agreed that the commuting schedule did not promote a healthy lifestyle and that it was interfering with their marital relationship. Frank again quit his old job and moved back to this community to be with his wife. He found a part-time job as a construction laborer. Unfortunately, the pay was considerably less than he had been making and he inwardly rebelled at taking orders instead of giving them.

His wife assured him her income was adequate for a

comfortable lifestyle for both of them and that she still respected him even though his job was a step down and his income half of hers. Her reassurances were apparently not adequate for his maintaining his sense of self-worth and he grew despondent. It was at this point that he arrived at my office with health fears, physical symptoms, and a feeling of desperation.

After obtaining some additional history from him, I established a diagnosis of andropause syndrome, but he was reluctant to accept it as a cause of his unhappiness and fatigue. I urged him to reconsider and suggested some reading material on male menopause. When he returned for his next office visit, there was no apparent improvement in his dysphoria or psychosomatic symptoms. He rejected my offer of a referral to a therapist and left the office saying he could work it out for himself. He returned to his home in the neighboring state, went back to work at his old job, and stopped commuting.

A year and a half later Frank and his wife filed for divorce.

Although it is good that we are moving toward a more equal society, there are several elements in the role reversal that impinge on the older male's ego. One must remember that today's mid-life man grew up in a society where male–female roles were more traditionally defined. Such a man's sense of self-importance is diminished when his wife brings home a larger paycheck. He becomes aware of his wife's reduced dependence on him as a provider. She spends more time away from home and less with him. Her interests expand beyond their home and relationship. Her work successes may outnumber his.

The andropausal man experiences as injurious a move to a different town to accommodate his wife's occupational demands. It's even more demeaning if he is unable to find satisfying work in the new location. *The Wall Street Journal* has labeled this pattern "the trailing spouse." The relationship and the man's self-esteem tend to deteriorate even further if the wife shows annoyance with her husband's relative decrease in monetary contribution to the household.

His loss of self-esteem produces unwelcome effects on the husband's mental and physical well-being. He often becomes defensive and miserable. Because the wife's independence impinges on his sense of masculinity, his sexual desire is likely to decrease. Often, destructive behavioral changes occur.

Wives seeking work out of the home in large numbers is a fairly new social phenomenon and illustrates how changing values in the industrialized world contribute to the andropausal condition. However, women will continue to play more and more important roles in the labor, business, and professional worlds. Men must make adjustments in their thinking and expectations to accommodate these changes. If they don't, they will be sentenced to ever-increasing resentment and unhappiness.

Fear of a destitute retirement can be one of the most troubling specters faced by those who approach old age. The middle-aged man who thinks about the future is apt to be troubled about the possibility of poverty, particularly if the financial goals he set for himself in his youth now appear to be out of his reach. Fear about security in old age can play a part in producing the psychological state of andropause. Careful and lifelong financial planning is obviously the best way to avoid this dilemma. There are many excellent publications on financial planning, so I'll leave this subject for the experts. There are, though, some observations about human nature and spending and saving which I feel are worth mentioning.

Everyone agrees that instituting a financial plan early in life is a good idea, but few people actually do so. It is, unfortunately, all too human to put off things until tomorrow, especially if the task is disagreeable and requires a change in lifestyle—saving instead of spending, for example.

The pleasures of spending sometimes override our better judgment. We are encouraged in spendthrift attitudes by advertising. A good deal of our spending is impulsive and excessive and we may find it easy to rationalize, telling ourselves, "I really need this," "I deserve the best," "This is a real bargain." Messages to ourselves simply echo the phrases of sales pitches we have heard.

We often expect to enjoy a standard of living that is too high to be maintained. An excessively high standard of living produces two fears: First, there is the fear that we will not have adequate funds in later life; second, there is the fear that we will not always be able to maintain the standard of living to which we have become accustomed. It is not easy to fight the tendencies to procrastinate so we ignore the future. The consequence of not saving is the fear of being poor when we are old. Andropausal men are not able to make mental adjustments to the realities of their financial condition.

o O o

Though it seems paradoxical, fear of old age and of death start very early in life. Even when we are only a few years old, experiences with death can leave us awed by its irreversibility. We may learn about death when a puppy gets run over or when a grandparent dies. Most of us have an early memory of our first or most strongly felt realization of death. As we grow older, we develop an awareness of the inevitability of the death of all things that live. Still, our own mortality usually remains incomprehensible. We push thoughts of it to the back of our minds and go about our lives as if we will live forever.

For men in mid-life, thoughts of death naturally start occurring more often. This is helpful to planning for their own deaths and for their survivors. However, in some men, apprehension about their eventual death becomes an obsession and can cause or aggravate andropausal symptoms.

Stress

Many self-help books currently on the market seem to address the issue of stress. Medically, stress is defined as the sum of the biological reactions to any adverse stimulus (physical, mental, emotional—internal or external) that disturbs a person's homeostasis, or normal balance. Stress happens within the body or mind in response to negative stimulation. Current usage of the word *stress* also includes the stimuli or stressors.

We are all exposed to stressors every day, but it is only when they reach an intolerable level (the threshold varies individually) that our bodies or minds react unfavorably. Until the last decade, the unfavorable reactions were usually termed anxiety or depression. Psychiatrists now use the term *adjustment disorder* when referring to stress reactions. The term *social adjustment* is used to indicate the skill of the individual in handling interpersonal situations.

Stressors can reach us in almost any setting—home, work, social. When our personal level of tolerance is exceeded, our minds, and frequently our bodies, react unfavorably. Anxiety is the most common reaction. We all have favorite nouns or adjectives to describe our own feelings of anxiety: nervous, uptight, raw nerves, upset, stressed out, etc. Recently, "burned out" has become a popular way to describe our reaction to stressors at work. The term usually indicates that there is some depression along with the anxiety.

Stress is also a factor in the andropause syndrome. All of the causal elements discussed in this chapter can be considered stressors, and the psychological changes that occur in male menopause could be described as stress. The anxiety and/or depression that results from stress can cause the viropause/andropause syndrome or aggravate an already existing condition. If the andropause has been caused by any of the other factors mentioned in this chapter, any concurrent stress-related anxiety will be intensified. To make matters worse, the mind of the andropausal man is less capable of sorting out and managing anxiety-producing stressors.

In our culture, stressors are forever increasing in number and force. In less industrialized areas, they are not accelerating as rapidly. But since we can't all move to a Greek island to reduce the stress in our lives, we need to learn to adjust to the pervasiveness of stressors. Adjustment strategies for the stress associated with andropause are discussed in Chapters 6 and 12.

Since medical research into male menopause is in its infancy, it's still not possible to identify the causes with any true scientific accuracy. However, observation of men experiencing the syndrome suggests the psychological causes include:

1. Unrealistic goals—goals that are too high or are otherwise unattainable;

2. Recognizing and rejecting the evidence of impairment of mind and body;

3. Changes in hormonal balance and sexuality;

4. Prospect of a decline in self-image that can occur at the time of retirement;

5. Fears about aging, displacement by wife, financial insecurity, illness, and death;

6. Stress.

My theory is that these probable psychological causes of male menopause are cultural byproducts; the more "civilized" the culture in which the man finds himself, the more likely he is to develop the condition. The likelihood of an individual experiencing male menopause varies. The greater the disparity between a man's expectations and reality, the more likely he is, in my opinion, to suffer from andropausal symptoms.

CHAPTER 5

Typical Reactions to Male Menopause

The transition from childhood to adulthood is not an easy one for adolescent boys. Their behavior tends to be erratic and emotional, but as a society we expect and understand this behavior. Just as there are similarities in the reactions of teenage boys to adolescence, there are similarities in men's emotional and behavioral reactions to viropause/andropause. The andropausal years are not smooth or easy either, but it comes as a surprise to spouses, families, and communities when men in their forties and fifties behave erratically and act out their emotional upheavals. We make allowances for teenage misdeeds, but not for the misdeeds of andropausal men. We believe implicitly that the transition to adulthood is a permanent change that heralds consistent behavior for the rest of a man's life. However, men's reactions to male menopause, we often believe, will continue whether we choose to acknowledge them or not.

Inadequacy, Anxiety, and Depression

A sense of personal inadequacy is a dominant component of male menopause. Understandably, the man who feels inadequate will look for ways to eliminate this unpleasant feeling. In our consumer-oriented society, many men experiencing the viropausal/andropausal syndrome respond in some fairly predictable ways that often include large expenditures in an effort to replace the perceived inadequacies in his life with purchases that he thinks will enhance his self-image. In andropause, a man has uncertainty about his worth and confusion about priorities so he is apt to make major decisions for the wrong reasons.

In addition to his feelings of inadequacy the andropausal man often suffers from feelings of anxiety. He usually assumes his anxiety is a response to external events or circumstances—a troubled marriage or problems at work—although he may not have an explanation for feeling tense. Regardless of what he perceives as the cause, he will try to find a way to relieve his anxiety because it doesn't feel good. A very common reaction to andropausal anxiety is using alcohol in increasing amounts to "unwind." Some men react by asking their doctors for tranquilizers and others resort to illegal drugs. Drug and alcohol abuse is quite common among andropausal men.

If the response to male menopause is a feeling of depression, the man who experiences it sometimes tries to escape that which he believes is the cause of his depression. For example, he may avoid certain people or places. A depressed man, like the anxious man, tends to use excessive amounts of alcohol or drugs, especially "uppers." The initial effect of alcohol is a feeling of euphoria that temporarily overrides the misery of depression. However, alcohol becomes a depressive after the first jolt, and coming down from drugs also produces depression, so the tendency is to take more in search of the temporary euphoria.

A distinction must be made between normal feelings of anxiety and the mental disorder of anxiety. All of us have an emotional response of anxiety in reaction to a consciously recognized internal or external threat or danger. For example, close airline connections cause most of us to feel anxious, but we would not be diagnosed with an anxiety disorder. For the menopausal man, anxiety is an emotional response to his fears and not a mental disorder. The same is true about feeling depressed as opposed to suffering from a depression disorder. Male menopause can easily be misdiagnosed as anxiety or depression disorders.

Andropause does sometimes coexist with anxiety or depression disorders. Each needs to be recognized and treated appropriately. This is not always easy because symptoms of each can overlap and appear similar. Medications are often useful in treating anxiety and depression disorders but are not usually indicated in the treatment of andropause.

There can be other significant mental reactions to male menopause. Sometimes the brain functions are altered so that attention and concentration decrease. This can impair a man's work performance and, if noticed, bring him angry responses from his boss or co-workers. If a man becomes aware of the changes, they add to his anxiety, depression, and fears and increase the severity of his andropause. He feels even more inadequate.

Behavioral Changes

The automobile is more than just a means of transportation. In America, and in many other countries, the automobile (or truck or motorcycle) is a symbol of power, masculinity, financial success, sexuality, superiority, and social or economic status. It's not surprising that andropausal men often purchase motor vehicles in order to relieve feelings of inadequacy or failure. A fast boat may be acquired for the same purpose. The choices are usually sporty or big and powerful. These vehicles are usually expensive, so the individual sometimes spends more than he can wisely afford. This extravagance may be a clue that this reaction is abnormal. (Young men also have a fondness for powerful, sporty cars. However, to them the cars represent maturity as well as power and masculinity.)

Gene Morgan had been fascinated by sports cars since his teen years. As soon as he could afford it, he bought an MG and for years was satisfied with owning a series of MGs. However, when he reached thirty-eight, he started yearning for a more powerful sports car.

It was about that same time that he started socializing with a circle of friends who were more affluent than he. His career was progressing as planned, but wasn't providing him a large enough income to allow him some of the luxuries his new friends enjoyed. The MGs he had always enjoyed no longer seemed adequate to his desires. He traded up for a red Jaguar.

He liked the Jag's fast acceleration, powerful braking system, and steering characteristics. He also particularly liked arriving at parties later than the other guests and making a spectacular entrance in his red "charger."

However, in another year or two, the Jag also starting seeming inadequate. Gene convinced himself that what he really needed was a more expensive (read impressive) car, so he traded up for a sporty Mercedes convertible. He felt temporarily satisfied but had twinges of anxiety every time he made his huge monthly payments.

When Gene eventually sought help for his increasing symptoms of male menopause, he was already starting to have some insight into his "hot rod" behavior. As counseling progressed, he was able to understand and accept that his car purchases were his way of compensating for feelings of inadequacy and lack of accomplishment.

Menopausal men may seek new friends who they believe to be of higher status—especially among the younger set. Those in a financial position to do so may order a larger and grander yacht. Others may accumulate additional residences in resorts like Palm Springs or on the Riviera. Still others may buy a baseball or basketball team.

Men who are running away from growing older by youth-seeking strategies are likely to be headed for trouble. A man who tries to buy back youth by spending extravagantly can find himself facing financial disaster. Automobiles, boats, jewelry, clothing, and vacations may temporarily bolster a man's ego, but they can also bring him and his family financial hardship or even ruin. When a man eventually realizes he has overspent, his anxiety increases and there is an accentuation of the feelings that led him to overspend in the first place. In extreme cases he may use illegal means to cover his debts.

Youthful Appearance

The normal deterioration of personal appearance—or perceived deterioration—becomes a matter of concern to the man in experiencing andropause. The degree of concern and response depends on how highly he values his bodily appearance. In response to the concern with their appearance, men may change their hair style, purchase a hairpiece or use color to cover up graying. Some may have transplants to balding areas or they may try one or more hair growth preparations. Some change their style of glasses. At all ages, both men and women select clothes to minimize what they see as unsightly lines of their bodies and maximize the attractive contours. As body lines deteriorate, appropriate clothing can camouflage the changes. The man experiencing male menopause tends to make some rather abrupt changes in his sartorial style. The menopausal male frequently selects clothing to portray a youthful appearance. In a culture that places high values on youth it is good business for clothiers to advertise youthful garments. Some men purchase jewelry such as neck chains, rings, or expensive watches. Some become clients of tanning facilities, believing a deeply tanned body is more youthful.

These attempts to reverse or camouflage the effects of time are common responses to male menopause, but these and other behavioral strategies are not effective in alleviating men's anxieties about growing old and may actually worsen their emotional health rather than easing the symptoms.

Men of all ages do things to try to reverse or retard the aging process. During male menopause, however, men are more likely to deny the evidence of aging or overcompensate for it. For example, they may attempt greater physical feats than ever achieved, even in their youth, or try to perform sexually at a superhuman level. Their goals for physical achievement may not be rational.

When a well-balanced older man sees signs of aging, he is more likely to accept them as a reality of life. His attempts to reverse or retard the changes are more rational. Instead of running faster and further, he may gear down to walking. He is more willing to accept the need for glasses than his andropausal counterpart. When the older man recognizes a decrease in his mental acuity, he is likely to take on less demanding or different tasks whereas the andropausal male may take on more difficult assignments in his effort to prove to himself and to others that he is still mentally sharp.

Reactions to aging in the psychologically sound older man are more likely to be reasonable, practical, and well-accepted. Reactions in the andropausal male are likely to be unreasonable, irrational and full of unrealistic or unattainable goals.

Health

The man experiencing viropausal/andropausal symptoms often becomes preoccupied with his health as well as with his physical appearance. He might engage in new physical activities, especially in sports where the young predominate. The need to have a younger self-image may be the motivating factor in starting an intense exercise program. It is generally agreed, of course, that physical exercise is healthy and desirable, but if the exercise is not appropriate to the age and physical condition of the individual, there may be deleterious effects. Participating in inappropriate new exercise may be a response to male menopause.

Late one afternoon I was called to the emergency room of the hospital to see one of my patients, Victor Lovett, who had been brought in by ambulance. A jogger had found him unconscious at the edge of the road on the outskirts of town. When he regained consciousness he told me that he was in the last mile of his weekly six-mile run and had felt lightheaded for about a minute, then could remember nothing until arriving at the hospital. He had experienced this symptom before while running and it always went away when he slowed his pace, so he had ignored it.

Three years previously, Victor had been given an electrocardiogram during an insurance examination. The physician told him then that he had a heartbeat irregularity and advised him to see his family doctor to have it further evaluated. Victor intended to follow the advice but never seemed to find the time. He wasn't too worried because the physician had added that it wasn't life-threatening.

Victor demonstrated a common reaction of the andropausal male: He refused to accept the possibility that he wasn't in perfect health. Men experiencing male menopause often consider a body deficit as an unacceptable and personal affront to their sense of adequacy and a threat to their self-esteem. Up to a point, that's normal, but overlooking conditions that cause any obvious disability or ignoring professional advice to have a condition investigated is abnormal or self-destructive behavior. During male menopause, a man's judgment is often impaired.

When Victor was forty-four, he began to develop dysphoria. Work was no longer satisfying, he was bored with his usual activities, and his home life was tedious. He became more and more sedentary and unhappy. A close friend of his who seemed exuberant about his own life was a regular jogger and often described the benefits of jogging. Victor concluded he should start an exercise program of his own.

He bought expensive and stylish running clothes and

started jogging twice a week. The first few weeks were tedious and disappointing, and Victor decided that the reason he wasn't experiencing the euphoria his friend did was that he wasn't exercising enough, so he increased the distance and the pace. Then he began noticing an excessive shortness of breath. Thinking it was because he needed more conditioning, he again stepped up the pace and distance. When he increased his distance from four to six miles, he began experiencing lightheadedness.

Victor came to me because he wanted a physical explanation for his dysphoria. He rejected a psychological explanation despite the fact that his symptoms were primarily mental and emotional. He also, typically, sought a quick fix for his negative feelings. This is understandable since health fad advertising tells us we can expect fast results with this or that food supplement or exercise.

Victor's hospital examination established a diagnosis of "sick sinus syndrome," which in some patients prevents an adequate cardiac response to exertion. On this occasion, Victor's heart hadn't pumped enough blood oxygen to his brain and he briefly lost consciousness.

Victor's hospital stay was short and I was able to treat him successfully for both his cardiac condition and male menopause symptoms in follow-up office visits. Both responded well to therapy.

Physical exercise is good for middle-aged men, but exercise that is not suitable for a particular individual can be harmful. Menopausal men, prodded by fears that their strength is declining and their masculinity threatened, are prone to embark on unrealistic programs of activities that are too vigorous and too strenuous. They often subscribe to the idea that if a little is good, a lot is better. A man who wants to show that he is still virile may try too hard to prove himself. The weights he lifts may be too heavy; the runs he makes may be too far or too fast. Moderate exercise is beneficial, but activity of more than customary vigor or duration can damage the skeletal system, especially that of an unconditioned body. For example, when the feet or knees are slightly misaligned, over-exercise can accelerate degenerative joint disease and thus actually worsen one of the physical manifestations of aging.

The sprains and strains that are common among sports participants heal more slowly with increasing age. Still more serious is the possibility that a middle-aged man's cardiovascular system may not be able to support the demands of unaccustomed physical activity. Exercise that is too strenuous can make the condition worse and can even lead to heart problems. We cannot always rely on our bodies to tell us when exercise is excessive or of the wrong type.

Physical and Psychosomatic Reactions

Though it is good for a person of any age to begin a physical exercise regimen, a physician's evaluation is recommended before starting a new program. Many men, however, are reluctant to have physical examinations. They may subconsciously believe that to admit they need one is a sign of weakness. Another possible reason so many men, especially men on the threshold of middle age, will not willingly have a physical examination is their fear that there may be something actually wrong with them. There are many other possible reasons, few of them sound, for not seeking medical advice about one's changing physical condition. The andropausal male, feeling especially vulnerable, is reluctant to admit his own limitations and is more likely than men of other ages to avoid getting a medical assessment of his physical condition. As a result, he may unwittingly harm himself.

The man experiencing menopause often develops psychosomatic health problems in addition to his physical signs of aging. These can vary considerably in character and severity and are usually their body's response to the anxiety component of the viropause/andropause syndrome. Psychosomatic reactions can be serious enough to be disabling, such as severe headaches, chronic indigestion, and abnormal heart rhythms. Because of the andropausal man's denial tendencies, the conditions often go undiagnosed and untreated. He may treat himself with over-the-counter medications like aspirin or antacids or he may use illegal drugs to suppress the symptoms.

Men experiencing menopause also react by gaining or losing weight. Men's eating habits can change in a variety of ways in reaction to stress; some men eat more and some eat less. Either way, a noticeable weight change in middle age is a probable sign of male menopause.

Reduced Sexuality

Reduced sexuality is a normal change in an aging man. When a man becomes aware of this, he is naturally concerned about it. After all, he has grown up in a society that equates sexuality with masculinity, power, and superiority. If the concern turns to worry and strong feelings of inadequacy, there frequently follows an unhealthy response. This sequence is common: The man becomes more aware of the younger females in his environment—maybe at work. He is flattered by any attention they may pay him. A friendship develops into a closer relationship and eventually includes sexual activity. Naturally, sex with a younger, different person is stimulating, so erectile powers are enhanced and libido increases. Consequently, the man feels more physically attractive, younger, and temporarily happier.

Some men at this point believe they have found "true love at last." They become unhappy with their wives and no longer find them attractive or sexually stimulating. They then may begin thinking of divorce and a new marriage. Unless this sequence is interrupted, divorce may ensue.

Robert Baker was a man who risked his marriage over an obsession with a younger woman. At age fifty-two, Robert appeared ill at ease when he arrived at my office. When he sat down he blurted, "I want an HIV test." When I asked why he explained, "I don't know why myself, but I've been cheating on my wife with another woman."

He went on to tell me that he had recently become friends with Jill, one of his co-workers. They started out discussing their mutual frustrations with management, but over a few weeks time, the conversations progressed to include personal matters. Robert was vaguely aware that perpetuating the relationship could lead to problems, but he asked Jill to go to lunch with him. They both felt uncomfortable, so they chose an obscure restaurant. The lunches soon became a weekly event.

Robert felt he had a good marriage, but the conversation at the lunches was stimulating and added excitement to his life. The clandestine meetings gave him a sense of adventure, and he felt exhilarated.

He explained that Jill was eleven years his junior, divorced, and had no children. He admitted that he was flattered that she sought his advice on personal and financial problems.

As the physical attraction grew, Robert found himself daydreaming about her body. He tried to put the erotic thoughts out of his mind, but failed. Eventually the couple planned a motel rendezvous in a neighboring town. According to Robert the afternoon was pure joy.

Men experiencing male menopause have lowered self-esteem and see themselves as less physically attractive, so they respond to someone who respects their mental acuity. Jill was young and attractive and paid special attention to Robert, which made him feel younger. She was also obviously impressed with his knowledge and experience, and he was pleased when she turned to him for advice. His feelings of inadequacy completely disappeared when he was with her.

They started meeting regularly at the motel and Robert was delighted with the return of his "real manhood." He noted his erections occurred spontaneously with very little stimulation and were harder. He found himself capable of two, sometimes three, orgasms in one afternoon. He was especially pleased with Jill's response to his physical needs. He compared his renewed sexuality to that in his marital relationship. In the preceding four years, his libido had been waning and he had thought that was "just natural for a man nearing fifty."

Early in an extramarital affair, the viropausal/andropausal man experiences a glorious feeling of recaptured youth. The negative feelings of inadequacy are eliminated and the perceived signs of aging seem to be reversed. However, the advantages are only temporary.

After five months of trysts, Jill took a leave of absence to be with her terminally ill mother in another state. It was during this time that Robert developed a case of remorse. He missed Jill terribly, but the more he missed her the more remorseful he became. The dysphoria of male menopause returned. Part of his remorse was really fear that he might have contacted AIDS from Jill and could have infected his wife.

On Robert's return visit to my office, he was much relieved to learn his HIV test was negative. I suggested he get some counseling to treat his viropausal/andropausal syndrome before he risked his health further.

Everyone, no matter what age, wants to feel attractive to members of the opposite sex. A man who is feeling the effects of age is more likely to seek love or sex in an extramarital affair than one who graciously accepts aging changes. Any romance can end unhappily, but an affair begun to allay a man's fears about aging is especially likely to. When a man is married and has a family, the potential for unhappiness is increased. If the man "recovers" from his infatuation, and even if his wife never learns of the affair, he may develop a sense of guilt that can scar his relationship with her. If his wife does learn of the affair, that, too, will change their relationship, undoubtedly for the worse. If the affair leads to divorce, then the breaking up of the family results in pain to everyone involved—the couple, the children, other relatives, and friends—everyone except the attorneys.

When there is a divorce and a new marriage to a younger wife, the andropausal man may not be realistic in his plans and hopes for the second marriage. If his expectations have been too optimistic, disillusionment progresses to misery and to regrets for him and his new wife. Men experiencing male menopause have distortions in their priorities and values and are not really competent to make important decisions about issues such as divorce and remarriage. Decisions should be delayed until there has been a recovery from the condition.

Emotional Changes

Typically, the viropausal/andropausal male is anxious, dysphoric, and fearful, and these feelings affect his behavior in ways that are often disruptive to his relationships. He troubles others with his irritability. He becomes impatient and angers easily. He overreacts to criticism and does not take kindly to suggestions from friends or family—especially suggestions about seeking professional help.

Another common viropausal/andropausal reaction is withdrawal. The man who recognizes his own irritability and fears saying things he might later regret withdraws to avoid possibly disastrous interactions with others. In his self-chosen solitude there are fewer reminders of the things that produce feelings of inadequacy and failure.

It's not pleasant being around an andropausal man who sees only the dark side of things. His tendency to talk about the unpleasant aspects of life—the world, the news, failures, death—makes him poor company. His dire predictions for the future, for himself, for his family, and for the world become tedious. A man's predominantly negative reactions to his male menopause can precipitate unfortunate and irreversible changes in his important relationships.

If a man recognizes, or is told that he has, symptoms of viropause/andropause, his first reaction will likely be one of rejection or denial. The reaction is similar to the reaction to loss. Whether it's loss of a friend, spouse or the possibility of andropause (loss of youth) there is a grieving process

that starts with denial: "No, this really isn't happening."
Then comes the anger: "I don't deserve this, it's somebody
else's fault, it's not fair." Next is acceptance: "Okay, this is
reality. What can I do about it?" And finally, there is adjustment, finding the means to go on with life despite the
feelings of loss.

A man's reactions to male menopause tend to be coun-
terproductive for himself and unsettling to his family and
friends. Hopefully his friends and family will recognize his
condition and be patient and supportive until he traverses
through and beyond this difficult period of his life. Their
efforts on his behalf will undoubtedly be appreciated in later years.

CHAPTER 6

Reducing the Impact of Andropause

Prevention of illness has advantages over treatment of illness. It's more effective to immunize against polio, for example, than to treat the disease; and most lung cancer can be prevented by not smoking. Preventative measures eliminate the threat of disease for some and greatly reduce the severity of symptoms in others. The prevention of psychological conditions also has a place in maintaining wellness, though it is somewhat more difficult to demonstrate. Modification of habits and lifestyle can prevent or reduce the severity and duration of andropause symptoms.

Obviously, the best way to prevent an illness is to remove the cause. Eliminating the cause of the male climacteric would be a reasonable approach to preventing the condition. If the causative factors cannot be removed, then an effort should be made to eradicate the precipitating factors. There are also ways to reduce the symptoms if the syndrome does occur.

CHAPTER 6

Goal Adjustments

Disappointment is one common cause of viropause/andropause—the disappointment a man experiences in midlife when he compares his earlier goals to his accomplishments thus far achieved. This disappointment trauma to the psyche is even more damaging when a man realizes there are limits to what he can still achieve in the remaining years of his life. Preventing or reducing the impact of male menopause requires a hard look at the realities governing our goals. This process can be painful for the man already suffering from male menopause.

The man who is "me"-motivated is highly susceptible to andropause. If his goals have been to accumulate money, status, and success, he is likely to experience the unhappiness of the male menopause. The illusion that wealth and status will give him happiness fades and leaves him with a sense of loss and a feeling of unworthiness.

When assessing achievements in relation to goals, the first category that comes to the mind of most men is financial success. Financial success is not about how much money is obtained but is related to future needs and is defined individually by each man. The only way a man can satisfactorily define it for himself is by relating it to his needs and not by comparing his financial status, favorably or unfavorably, with that of anyone else.

A man experiencing viropausal/andropausal symptoms is likely to think of financial success in relative terms. No doubt almost every man could improve his financial position, at least to some degree, with additional effort and striving. But the costs may be too high. Such costs could be the impairment of personal relationship or the erosion of health through physical exhaustion or the anxiety of stress.

Vague ideas about how much is needed may lead to worry, frustration, and anxiety. To avoid such frustration, most of us need some professional help in making financial plans. With such help most individuals can realistically decide what will truly give them contentment in later life——hobbies, traveling, and so forth. It is helpful to develop rather definite ideas about these matters. However, it is also important not to feel compulsive about the fixed amounts. Appropriate modifications from time to time should be expected and acceptable.

To avoid contracting andropause, men would be wise to review and realistically modify their financial and other goals during their twenties and thirties. They might ask themselves: Is this goal what I really want or need, or is it reflecting someone else's desires? If it's not what I want, what do I really need to be happy? Are my goals realistic? Are they attainable? If not, what goals are realistic and attainable? Modifications are not failures but rather reality adjustments that will better promote a personal sense of achievement and happiness. Even the modifications are not static. Goals need to be re-evaluated and changed from time to time as our lives change.

Learning to accept the need for such changes can be a tedious and, at times, an unpleasant part of the process of managing one's life. But designing and accepting realistic goals will prevent one of the major causes of andropause: disappointment.

When a man experiencing male menopause recognizes that it is futile to seek happiness through the accumulation of money, objects, and status, he has taken a step toward achieving recovery. The next step he could take might be to take an inventory of himself. The man with viropausal/

andropausal symptoms should analyze what is inside himself. If he finds things that he doesn't like, he should plan to take action to eliminate them. The list of changes he wants to make in himself may be very long, or it may be short. He may find that he wants to eliminate dishonesty, selfishness, greed, and vanity. His self-inventory should also reveal qualities in himself which can be seen as assets, such as generosity, honesty, and a loving, caring nature. He should allow himself to appreciate these qualities, and he may want to enlarge upon them.

Writing down observations about goals is more effective than making mental notes. A list can provide more precise and useful material on which to base conclusions. Written thoughts should be secret and destroyed after they have served their purpose, not saved for the future, or they may not be honestly recorded.

The first step is making a list of the initial goals established in earlier years. For most men this means thinking back to high school and college days. Then add to the list modifications made in those goals in the subsequent years. The list should include intellectual achievements, development of personal relationships, and community status, as well as physical and financial successes. Determine if these goals were reasonable and realistic.

The second step is making a list of goals for the future. Being honest, indicate and define future goals that are realistic. What is in the realm of possibility? What is truly reachable during the remainder of your life span? Expect this step to take some time. It will require a close look at others in the world and considerable thought and should include the prioritization of goals. It helps to acknowledge that future goals may have to be modified as time passes.

Estimates of future goals may be too high or too low. They will require fine tuning from time to time.

Step three is the mental and emotional acceptance of the adjusted goals. By acknowledging the world as it is rather than inventing an impossible world he would like, a man can value his true accomplishments and avoid disappointment.

The outcome of the goal adjustment program should be positive self-esteem in relationship to goals. It is almost impossible to prevent or recover from andropause without developing an acceptable and realistic self-image.

Retirement

Few young men consider their eventual retirement as they enter the work world. The event is so far in the future that they dismiss it from their minds. But plans for retirement should be included in their life planning. Those who think ahead and make retirement part of their scheme are less likely to succumb to the male menopause.

At the time of retirement, men consciously or subconsciously reevaluate their lives including their financial position, social status, and self-image. The end of a lifelong occupation is often disruptive and can precipitate a significant reduction in self-esteem.

Planning for a second occupation or avocation that helps maintain a sense of self-worth is one way to avoid the dissapointments of retirement. Several years before his anticipated retirement, a man should select a second interest and develop it. For many men the choice will be an interest that has been a lifetime hobby. For others it might be a totally new avenue of endeavor. It must, in any case, be some activity that supports self-esteem.

Many men who retire look forward to doing things they did for fun on their days off—hunting, fishing, or golfing, for example. Others are anxious to get to jobs that they have neglected—clean the garage, fix up around the house, and so on. These are certainly worthwhile activities and should be included in a retirement plan. Unfortunately, enthusiasm for these tasks sometimes wanes, and retirees find time heavy on their hands. At this point they may feel they've become second-class citizens, especially if they have nothing of importance to fill their time.

Activities requiring physical vigor may not always be the best choice. As a man ages, his mind stays vigorous longer than his body, so pursuits of an intellectual nature may be more suitable. Some men find managing their own investments exciting and rewarding. Others return to college to rediscover "old loves" such as art, music, or literature.

There are many, many, enjoyable ways to occupy one's time in retirement years. Scores of books are available on the subject. There are organizations that specialize in helping retired people find interesting activities. It is most important to select one or more interests early and get started before retirement day. The first one chosen may not be suitable. If the process of developing leisure time interests is started long before retirement, there's time to change or add new ones.

Not everyone retires, but in some occupations retirement is forced and working beyond a certain age is not permitted. Such is true of public servants who are appointed rather than elected, members of the teaching profession, career athletes, and professional members of the military. (In the 1980s, for financial reasons, large companies developed new retirement programs. Early retirement was encouraged in order to replace more highly paid, older employees with lower paid, younger employees.) Generally, it is the self-employed who find they can continue to work beyond the usual retirement age.

The early choice of occupation determines whether or not retirement programs affect later life. When young men choose their lifetime occupations they usually look at the satisfaction and financial benefits provided by the occupations considered. Rarely do retirement factors enter into their decisions. However, the last twenty or thirty or more years of their lives are influenced greatly by these very early decisions. Having a viable plan for retirement can help prevent or reduce the impact of andropause by relieving the stress or anxiety about the unknown future.

Physical Aging

All men experience some of the physical and mental changes common to aging, but all men do not experience clinical male menopause. However, some men's emotional reaction to the changes of aging is a component of the syndrome. The andropausal male has a poor self-image and this often generalizes to include his physical appearance. He dislikes what he sees in the mirror and does not have a feeling of vigor. By doing all that he can to improve his physical condition, he will improve his self-image and diminish the effects of male menopause.

One aspect of our self-esteem is how we perceive our bodies and our health. We are bombarded these days by sports and fitness shows that emphasize the many benefits of vigorous physical activity. The man experiencing male menopause feels inferior when assessing his own state of health. In comparison, there is always someone his age with a stronger, more agile body.

One's middle years are an excellent time to take inventory. "Could I look and feel better? Is it possible for me to become more physically fit? Is fitness important to me? Are the time, effort, and cost worth it to me?" Some men never achieve optimal fitness unless they participated in school sports or were in some branch of the military service. For these men, an effective fitness program can produce a new high and can be a powerful therapeutic element in the recovery from male menopause.

After he has done everything reasonable to improve his physical health, a man must learn to accept the remaining imperfections. Physical disabilities that resist correction, such as arthritis or a back injury or a heart condition, need special consideration. The man in andropause must accept that which cannot be changed. He must then learn to accommodate these deficiencies in both his thinking and his activities.

There are numerous articles, books, and videotapes on the subjects of healthy diets and exercise, so I will not attempt to enlarge on these subjects except to say that a proper diet and adequate, appropriate exercise are fundamentally important to a man's mental outlook and energy level.

A less discussed subject is that of plastic surgery as a means to improve physical appearance. Facial contours are an important physical element of a man's self-image. For many years women have recognized this fact and have taken appropriate steps to improve the appearance of their faces. Men have been reluctant to take these steps; they have a mind set that it's not masculine to have a face lift.

Not all men are candidates for facial plastic surgery. It can improve a man's appearance, but it can't change his personality. It won't cure male menopause. However, for the andropausal male whose primary symptom is anxiety about the appearance of aging, and who can afford it, plastic surgery can serve a useful purpose in the process of recovery.

Even though it may not always make them look older, men do not like losing their hair. Balding can be a precipitating factor in the onset of the male climacteric, though not a direct cause. There are some effective prescription lotions available that help retard hair loss and possibly encourage regrowth.

Men who have allowed their bodies to deteriorate are at high risk to develop the viropause/andropause syndrome. A word of caution is in order. Do not expect to achieve the level of fitness experienced in the teens and twenties. Use good judgment and be realistic.

At fifty-nine, Vincent Reynolds's judgment was not very good. I saw him in the hospital emergency room with a spiral fracture to his ankle. He had fallen while skiing on the local slope.

Vince had taken up skiing the previous year after a life of very little physical activity, but because of his eagerness he had learned quickly. One of his ski instructors had told him to "attack the mountain," and that advice dominated his subsequent skiing style. His friends called him "the wildman on skis."

He started the ski season without any pre-season training exercises. He preferred to get in shape on the slopes. He was always one of the first ones on the lifts and the last to take off his skis. He had been told by an instructor that it was best to stop for the day when fatigue set in, but he ignored this advice and continued for another hour or two after his legs were noticeably tired and slower to respond.

There was no significant displacement of bones at the fracture site, so only a cast was needed. Follow-up visits revealed no other physical problems except that he had slowed down a bit. Vince reported a feeling of decreased well-being. His work was less stimulating and he took longer lunch breaks with one or two martinis. He felt sluggish in the afternoons so he often went home from work earlier. He and his wife were divorced, and he was alone in the evenings. He was gradually increasing his liquor intake and the evening meal was nutritionally inadequate.

During the visits for his ankle injury, various aspects of male menopause were discussed. Vince readily accepted the concept and began appropriate reassessment of his goals and priorities. During our last visit, we discussed how to enjoy skiing with lower risks including pre-season conditioning, how to recognize fatigue that increases the chance of injury, and sticking to terrain that was not too difficult for his skiing skills. I advised him not to use the sport to prove to himself that he was still a young man, but rather to use it as a way to enhance the quality of his life despite some aging changes in his body. His leg healed well and he was back on skis the following season, a much wiser skier.

Some aging changes can be eliminated, some can be modified, some can be retarded or delayed, and some we cannot control. One way to retard the effects of aging is to avoid hazardous habits that are likely to damage body organs and structures, for example, smoking cigarettes, which produces skin wrinkling and reduced physical endurance. Developing good health habits early in life is an important

part of preventing serious symptoms of the male menopause syndrome.

Self-Esteem

Some of the seeds of the viropause/andropause syndrome can be sown during childhood. For example, feelings of self-worth are a product of one's experiences during
the first several years of life. Low self-esteem in mid-life is
associated with male menopause. Positive self-worth is the
essential requirement for happiness. Unless we accept ourselves as we are, we will spend our lives trying to prove
that we are worthwhile by actions that will leave us feeling
empty and in relationships that are doomed to failure. In accepting ourselves, we set aside any need to impress ourselves or others.

Self-esteem implies the ability to see our own good-
ness, appreciate our talents and accomplishments, and cele-
brate our humanness; it implies an acknowledgment our
uniqueness and specialness. One of the most predominant
symptoms of the andropausal man is his lack of contentment with who he is and what he has achieved.

For the young, happiness reflects being involved in a
parade of fun, a continuous whirl of activities and excitement. When there is a pause between episodes of excitement, young people may say, "I'm bored." As they grow
older and wiser, they come to realize that happiness is
something more than taking part in fun activities. Unfortunately, not everyone develops this wisdom easily or automatically. When the activities slow, they feel discontented,
and for men, this discontentment may lead to andropause.

In our society it is remarkably easy to accept the idea
that happiness is a result of possessing things of monetary

value: clothes, houses, cars, money in the bank, a solid investment portfolio. In short, happiness appears to be something that can be purchased by those who are affluent. However, we all know, whether consciously or unconsciously, that joy doesn't come from affluence but from our feelings of self-worth and self-acceptance and from happy and compatible relationships with those about us.

Possessions are indeed desirable for comfort, and we humans are creatures who like comfort. Financial assets are definitely needed to provide, among other things, shelter and food, but they have little to do with our feelings of self-acceptance. Unfortunately, our self-image often develops as a comparative concept. We may value ourselves according to how we appear to ourselves in comparison to other people we admire or compare what we have to what they have. Contentment is not a comparative feeling. There is always going to be someone who has more or is better. Once the man experiencing male menopause accepts himself, he no longer needs to impress others or fear their achievements in relation to his own. Taking this step to accept oneself is very important in the treatment of andropause, and sometimes this step requires outside guidance.

A patient, Keith Daniels, fifty-eight, called and asked if I would suggest some books he could read on the subject of male menopause. He had read my most recent medical column in the local newspaper, which had been about andropause. He explained that if he could read up on the subject he could probably handle his problems without counseling. I was inclined to agree with him. I knew Keith as a friend as well as a patient, and he was an intelligent, resourceful, well-balanced man.

When he came to my office, I was shocked by his

general appearance; in contrast to his usually buoyancy, he was sober and hardly smiled. I gave him a list of three books I thought might be helpful and apologized for not having better references. There are no good publications in print that deal exclusively with male menopause. Keith thanked me for what I gave him and agreed to my suggestion that we have a talk after he finished the books.

About three weeks later, Keith returned the books and said he needed to talk about his own andropause. He appeared haggard and was somewhat restless. Without preliminary chatting or delay, he described his symptoms and what he thought the causes were.

He had become depressed eight months earlier, soon after he and his wife had returned from a visit to an old college friend in another state. He and his friend had graduated together with degrees in business administration and had shared a room in the fraternity house the last two years of college. They had often discussed their goals and their plans for the future. From my friendship with Keith, I knew he was now a successful businessman and had good relationships with his family.

Soon after graduation his friend found employment in a growing firm, got some good breaks, and moved up to a top executive position. His success was evident in his opulent home in a pricey neighborhood. On previous visits, Keith had been vaguely aware of the disparity in their financial success, but on this last visit, he had become acutely aware of it. He found himself recalling his own goals and started depreciating his own accomplishments. He tried to tell himself that he made a comfortable living and had a wonderful family and many good friends, but it didn't help. His unhappiness intensified.

After discussing some other symptoms, Keith and I agreed that he was indeed experiencing male menopause and turned to what steps he could take to achieve recovery. We talked about goal adjustments, maintaining a healthy body, lifestyle modification, and reordering priorities. I suggested a quiet retreat by himself to do some quiet thinking. A week later he called to tell me he had taken a week off and had reservations at a monastery operated by his church. I offered him some guidelines to direct his thoughts during the retreat and we said goodbye.

When Keith returned, he called to report that the quiet days had done him "a world of good" but admitted he had a long way to go before he would be fully recovered. After that, I saw him occasionally at social events and he would briefly report he was doing better.

Seven months later, Keith came in for his annual physical and told me that, following the guidelines we had set up to combat his symptoms of andropause, he had really turned his life around. He was finding a new kind of satisfaction in his business, and he and his wife were starting to make travel and activity plans for their retirement in seven years. At home, he was drinking less and enjoying more energized sexual activity with his wife. They were much closer and seemed to have more to talk about, and they had started entertaining old friends again. With his restored self-esteem, Keith found the slightly slower pace a delightful change, and his life had new meaning. He was happily looking forward to his next visit with his college friend.

One approach to self-treatment for the man in viropause/andropause is to stop and think about what is best for himself instead of what is best for others. A contented man benefits all who come in contact with him as well as himself. But self-acceptance doesn't imply perfection or completion. There may still be many things that need changing. Whatever they are, large or small, if they are changes that will increase self-contentment, this is the time to begin them. Before beginning, however, it is important to remember that we cannot change others, only ourselves.

A useful approach to self-assessment is to try to see oneself as others do—family, fellow workers, community. To start the evaluation, a man might try to imagine what thoughts others would have about him if he were to die at this moment. Beyond the immediate reaction of grief, how would the people in his life remember him? How would they feel about his absence? If the answers aren't satisfactory, there is still time to make some changes.

The middle years offer most men more time to spend with their families. Commonly, men in their earlier years feel forced to spend much of their time meeting the demands of work, financial needs, and the desire for security. Many men experiencing male menopause feel guilty about having neglected their families earlier, so the time now spent with them can alleviate some of these feelings.

In our society, time has great value. In a sense we have become slaves to time—to clocks, to schedules, and to deadlines. Rather than becoming overwhelmed by the time that is slipping away from them, andropausal men must free themselves from this slavery by reassigning priorities for the use of their time. One of the ways they can do this is by sharing some of their time with a younger man.

The word *mentor* is taken from the name of the man who gave his advice and wisdom to the young son of Odysseus. A careful study of history will show that immense contributions have been made by aging men who undertook the guidance and assistance of a younger man. At the age of sixty-one, Plato became the seventeen-year-old Aristotle's mentor, then young Alexander learned from Aristotle when Aristotle grew older. One means of achieving the transition necessary to bring an end to male menopause may be to undertake the task of becoming a mentor and choosing a protégé.

Our overvaluing of time has conditioned us to hurry and to be impatient with delay. Men who are in their middle years may have difficulty slowing down and learning to be patient. But it is important for them to do so. It is less necessary for them to rush than it may have been in the past. Though occasionally decisions must be made without delay, they are best made after a period of calm deliberation. Most men, as they mature, grow to recognize the folly of impatience and of hasty decisions. The man experiencing male menopause, though, continues to hurry through day-to-day life. The hurrying is likely to result in tension and to produce feelings of anxiety. The anxiety in turn causes irritability and poor judgment, which are two common signs of andropause.

Men suffering from the viropause/andropause syndrome step closer to recovery when they develop the habit of patience. The individual who wants to stop being impatient can begin by taking the time to look realistically at his habits. He can make adjustments in his time priorities. It may take effort to learn to slow down, so he should not be in a hurry to achieve this goal. Not only does taking time to reach decisions produce respect in others, patient introspection is also conducive to self-respect. Priorities fall into place better when one allows them time to do so.

Facing the Fear of Death

The fear of death seems to be an intrinsic part of our psyches and must be considered a normal emotional reaction to the unknown. Every person who lives faces that fear, but when thoughts of death take over and become obsessive, they are abnormal. If the fears occupy the mind for long periods of time, create deep and lasting unhappiness, alter behavior radically, or are destructive to relationships, they are abnormal. Frequently, whether consciously acknowledged or not, an obsessive fear of death is part of the andropausal syndrome.

Fear of death starts very early in life. To avoid the psychic trauma that it can induce in mid-life, it helps to begin thinking about death early in the twenties or thirties. This need not be a gloomy experience but rather a time to discover one's own resources and strength. When one realistically confronts the idea of death, new attitudes and ideas can develop—ones that are more acceptable. A philosophy (wisdom and knowledge) can replace fear and feelings of discomfort. Adjusting to unpleasant realities is difficult but necessary to reach a state of contentment.

There is no single way to remove the fear of death, no approach that will work for everyone. Dealing with it adequately may require professional help for some. But there are some self-help measures that have been found to be useful.

Accepting one's own mortality and getting used to it is a slow process. For many people the study of religion provides a way of dealing with their fear of death. Most religions concern themselves, at least in part, with what happens after death. Religious study, even the comparative study of different religions' points of view about death, may offer guidance.

The study of secular philosophy is another non-religious approach to dealing with these fears. The great thinkers confronted mortality just as the rest of us do, and their insights can prove rich and profound.

Reviewing aspects of psychology may also afford insights that can prove helpful. Human beings alone have thoughts of their own dissolution, and psychologists have found this human concern a particularly relevant field for their investigations.

Making definitive plans for one's death can be a useful exercise. For a man experiencing greater fear of death due to viropause/andropause, it helps to confront one's own death realistically. Most people think of their death in vague terms, then when forced by a life threatening illness they are devastated and often it is too late to make a smooth transition from vague thoughts to realistic acceptance. Preparing and filing a will is advisable both for legal reasons and for developing greater awareness of one's eventual death. As financial circumstances change, the will can be updated, serving as a reminder of the eventual termination of life. Other planning such as deciding between cremation and burial, which cemetery, and the distribution of possessions not included in the will are useful for the same reasons. The decisions should be written out and discussed with family members.

It might seem that thinking about one's own death would be depressing, but in fact it often decreases feelings of depression. Planning and making decisions eliminate some of the unknowns ahead, which reduces feelings of anxiety.

Though it may seem unbelievable to those who are

young and to the viropausal/andropausal man who is deeply troubled by the fear of death, the fear does lessen with age. Men between the ages of forty and fifty-five are much more intensely concerned about death than they will be at seventy. One would guess that the closer a man comes to the end of life, the more preoccupied he would become with it. In reality the reverse is true. For most men, old age brings a diminution in the fear of death. In spite of its presumed closeness, it is not at the forefront of their minds. Perhaps it is another example of the human mind's capacity to gradually adjust to the inevitable.

Setting Priorities

In his book *Essays in Disguise*, Wilfred Sheed describes the twenties of a man's life as "the decade . . . in which reality begins in earnest to crowd out imagination." The forties appears to be the decade in which the past begins to crowd out the future. For younger men, the promise of the future influences their self-image. They are, they believe, what they have the potential to become. In their andropausal years, men are forced to accept the fact that their potential has, for the most part, already been realized. The andropausal man finds this acceptance difficult, or maybe even impossible. The consequences of nonacceptance are anxiety and depression. No matter how painful, reordering priorities for the second half of life is necessary for recovery from the andropausal condition. What was most important at twenty or thirty years of age will almost certainly be different from what is most important at forty and beyond.

Men in their menopausal years often become uncomfortable with their established priorities. This discomfort may be one of the factors that determine whether or not a particular man will succumb to andropause or how severely he will be affected.

During the teen years, and then again during mid-life, what a man regards as important undergoes abrupt and significant change. The rapid change can be disquieting and the resulting confusion can lead to behavioral changes as well. At the end of the menopausal years, men again move into a state of maturity which does not refer to old age, but to an improved mental state, often referred to as self-actualization (a word coined by therapist Abraham Maslow in 1954).

The man experiencing male menopause should be aware that it is natural for his priorities to change at this time in life. It is worthwhile to review and change priorities until he is satisfied that his are the right ones to sustain his feeling of well-being. He must continue to evaluate and rearrange his priorities until they are suitable for him during the next decades of life.

Priorities may be categorized according to a variety of systems. Here is one list of categories that can be used as a guide to get started.

1. Human relationships (intangibles): family, friends, acquaintances at work and other places, members of the community;

2. Possessions (tangibles): wealth, assets, investments, primary home, secondary homes (RVs), items of transportation (cars, boats, yachts, planes, motorcycles), jewelry;

3. Activities: communication with others, hobbies, travel, leisure and pastime activities, educational pursuits, religious endeavors.

One priority change that I see frequently in men experiencing male menopause is a desire to change residence. Early in life men strive to own a suitable home for themselves and their families. Later, especially after the children are grown, a large home becomes a burden, so they sell it and purchase a smaller home or condo. The small home becomes a stopover between trips and other activities. On the other hand, some men continue to place a high priority on their family home and spend their andropausal years doing maintenance and making improvements that help fulfill their changing needs for contentment.

Though there are many ways to reduce the impact of male menopause, it is an unhappy state for most men and it is unrealistic to expect a sudden return of happiness. Though men are impatient by nature, they generally realize that most of the important events in life cannot be hastened. Though we can be persuaded by the "credit card mentality" to expect to get some things now, there are things, maturity has taught us, for which we must wait. Patience is a virtue more easily practiced as we grow older. So the man who has undertaken the task of helping himself through viropause/andropause should make adjustments in his thoughts and behavior and then exercise patience in waiting for signs of recovery. It may come in a few days—some experiences or insights may produce sudden changes. For most of the men who are experiencing male menopause, such changes will take weeks or months.

CHAPTER 7

Female Menopause and Sexuality

One of the purposes of this book is to present information about the possible problems, including the sexual changes, that men in their viropausal/andropausal years may experience. Women also change at this time in their lives, physically, emotionally, and sexually. Because a man's climacteric (change of life), as it relates to sexuality, often comes at the same time as his wife's, a brief discussion of female menopause is appropriate.

Not too long ago, most women dreaded the approach of menopause because they believed it to be a time of life when their femininity and sexuality diminished—a time of desexualization. More recently, this point of view has undergone change. Benefiting from sociological and medical research, education, the women's movement, and mass media communication, there are women who now see menopause as the phase in their lives when sexuality *increases*. Several explanations have been offered for this increase: no fear of pregnancy and no need for contraception, no inconvenience of menses, fewer responsibilities (such as child care), more time to spend on themselves, more self-assurance, a realization that sexual attraction is not just physical, and changes in hormonal balance. Also, as the hormone estrogen decreases in middle-aged women, their adrenal glands (glands above the kidneys that secrete hormones) play a more dominant role, and this increases libido.

Menopause and Andropause

Menopause literally refers to the date of the first missed menses, but the term is now commonly used to represent the period of time in which a multitude of physical and psychological changes take place. A woman's last menses normally occurs some time between forty-five and fifty-five but may be as early as thirty-eight. In comparison, male menopause typically starts in the forties or fifties, but it also can occur in the late thirties.

The duration of both female menopause and male menopause is variable. The average span of menopausal symptoms is three to five years, but can be as short as a few months or as long as ten years. Female menopausal symptoms can be reduced by the use of estrogen or other medications. Lifestyle can also alter the duration. In general, good mental and physical health habits shorten menopause and decrease the severity of symptoms.

The major difference between male and female menopause is hormonal. Almost universally, the decrease and eventual end of gonadal (ovarian) hormone production in women plays a major role in their menopausal symptoms, whereas the gradual reduction of male hormone (testosterone) is rarely a significant factor in andropausal symptoms. In men the decrease is minimal until age sixty, and very few men ever suffer a total absence of testosterone.

Men and women experiencing menopause have different behavioral reactions to their experiences. Women are much more likely to accept the realities of the changes brought on by menopause, to make the necessary mental and emotional adjustments, and to seek professional help for their symptoms. Men tend to deny their andropausal symptoms or seek superficial and ineffective "quick fixes" for them. Though many women pass through their menopausal years with symptoms so slight they don't need medical attention, there is a small percentage with extreme symptoms who do need professional assistance. Some, like my patient Cicely Fulsom, are urged into getting help by their husbands.

At the close of her husband Alan's annual physical, I asked the usual question: "Is there anything else you would like to talk about?" He looked a bit uncomfortable and paused before answering. Finally he said, "No, there isn't, at least about myself, but if it's okay, I'd like to ask about my wife." I assured him he was welcome to discuss any problems his wife was having, as his wife's health affected his health and well-being also.

Cicely was fifty-one and, according to her husband, seemed to have had a "personality change." She had become irritable and at times unreasonable. Alan was concerned about her physical health as well. She was having trouble sleeping and consequently was lethargic during the day. I asked Alan if his wife was having hot flashes. He didn't think she was, but mentioned that several nights during the past six months they had gotten up to change the bed after her perspiration had drenched the sheets.

I told Alan that his wife may have entered menopause, but that other physical conditions could produce the same pattern of symptoms. I advised that she get a physical examination and some tests. He agreed, and the next day his wife called to schedule a time.

When Cicely arrived for her appointment, she seemed slightly annoyed and told me, "I want you to know this was my husband's idea, not mine." However, after several minutes of conversation, she relaxed and began to describe her symptoms and past medical history accurately.

The symptoms were fairly classic for early menopause. Beginning one year earlier her menstrual periods became irregular, then stopped completely six months later. Concurrently, she started experiencing insomnia, night sweats, and occasional hot flashes. She was aware of becoming short-tempered and felt guilty for letting her husband see it. She offered an explanation—her oldest daughter was having some problems with her pregnancy. She apologetically added, "I guess I've become a real worrier."

During the history-by-systems, she also revealed a sexual problem: She had become less interested in sex and would avoid it when she could think of a reasonable excuse, partly "because intercourse is sometimes painful." The last few times she and her husband had used a lubricant, which had helped reduce the pain.

A week later we sat down together and discussed the physical findings and laboratory results, and I explained to her my diagnosis of early menopause with estrogen deficiency. I gave her some material to read on both subjects and suggested she ask her husband to read it also. I also gave her a prescription for estrogen and Progestin (synthetic progesterone) tablets. We discussed a cyclic program for their use, and I asked her to keep a record of the vaginal bleeding that would occur as part of each cycle as a reaction to the hormone tablets. We scheduled a return visit in two months.

On her return visit, Cicely seemed happier and more at ease than on previous visits. She reported an improvement in her sleeping habits and had no more night sweats. The pain of intercourse had eased, and she was becoming more positive about her sexuality. She expressed amazement at how quickly (less than a week) the improvements had occurred after she started on the estrogen tablets. She ended by saying she was feeling better than she had for months.

At Christmas time, I received a card from Alan and his wife expressing their thanks, and I noted that both Alan and Cicely had signed it.

Symptoms of Menopause

There are many more physical symptoms common to female menopause than to male menopause. As ovary activity decreases and estrogen production is reduced, certain physical changes occur. One in particular interferes with normal sex activity—vaginal dryness. The troublesome dryness of the vaginal lining is very common during menopause. Significantly, it is often the first sign of estrogen deficiency. Contrary to common belief, hot flashes are not the herald of menopause, but rather it is the inadequacy of moisture in the vagina that signals the onset of menopause. This fact is usually not recognized by women, and even some physicians are unaware of it.

During sexual excitement the vaginal mucosal lining produces a large amount of slippery, clear fluid. It has the same physical characteristics as the liquid that flows from the male urethra during sexual excitement before ejaculation. The amount of the fluid that is produced varies throughout the life of the female. Teenage girls produce a profuse flow during sexual arousal. It takes relatively little sexual excitement at this time of sexual life to start the process. As the years pass, the amount of liquid produced gradually decreases and more stimulation is required to start the flow. In the early menopausal years, the flow becomes minimal regardless of the sexual stimulation.

I suspect that the reason less is known about this symptom than about hot flashes is because women are not inclined to discuss it with their friends, nor are they likely to mention it to their physician. It is only when I ask a direct question, "Do you have dryness of the vagina during intercourse?" that my patients report the problem to me. Women then are likely to tell me of the difficulties with intromission (insertion of the penis into the vagina) and their discomfort. Often their pain is enough to interfere with sexual function, and they will not achieve orgasm. It is difficult to have a desire for sex and affectionate feelings when there is vaginal pain during intercourse. Patients who are experiencing these symptoms are relieved when I tell them the condition is reversible—curable—with the use of low-dose estrogen which can be orally or vaginally applied.

The subject of dryness in the vagina may seem inappropriate in a book on male menopause, but men should be aware of it. A man may feel inadequate and fear that he is no longer sexually attractive to his partner because she does not achieve orgasm. If he understands that the real problem could be vaginal dryness and the pain it can cause, he does not have to blame himself. Both partners should both understand the problem can easily be solved.

This provides an example of why communication is vital to a good sexual relationship. Conversation helps clarify problems: "Darling, I'm sorry it's taking so long for me to come, but tonight your penis is hurting me." "I'm sorry you're having pain, but I'm relieved to know it. I was thinking maybe I wasn't turning you on." One solution is to use an artificial lubricant. Many choose the inexpensive petroleum jelly, but others prefer to use one of the water-soluble lubricants, because they are easily wiped away or washed off after intercourse.

Vaginal pain can also be caused by the shrinking of the vagina which occurs in some women sometime after menopause. The shrinkage can make intromission painful and difficult. The shrinkage can be retarded by taking estrogen. However, it is less likely to occur if the woman engages in sexual intercourse regularly. The erect penis helps to keep the entrance to the vagina dilated. This can also be accomplished with a dilatory device, which is obtainable from medical suppliers with a physician's prescription.

Hot flashes are almost synonymous with menopause for many women. Estrogen controls the "thermostat" centers that constrict or dilate the small blood vessels near the surface of the skin that keep the skin at an even temperature. When estrogen decreases during menopause, the system malfunctions and the skin overheats. Night sweats are also a manifestation of this malfunction. Another menopause symptom, insomnia, may also be connected to the thermostat malfunction. It's possible that women are sub-

CHAPTER 7

consciously aware of the frequent changes in their skin
temperature and this awareness disturbs their sleep.

Hormonal Changes

The ovarian production of hormones—estrogen beginning during menses and progesterone during ovulation—affect a woman physically, emotionally, and sexually
although there is no scientific consensus regarding the effects of these hormones on libido and responsiveness. Some
women reach the pinnacle of their libido after their
menstrual period, others during ovulation, and still others
during the few days before menses.

The release of estrogen contributes to a woman's feeling of well-being while the release of progesterone is associated with depression in some women. Synthetic
progesterone is often prescribed to alleviate symptoms of
PMS (premenstrual syndrome) but the associated side effects of depression and increase of cholesterol and triglycerides can be worrisome.

If ovulation does not occur (common during the pre-
menopausal years), menstrual patterns change. Menses may
occur earlier or later, and the amount of blood loss can vary
with periods, even being skipped for a few months. Since
there is no release of progesterone when there is no ovulation, it is possible that PMS symptoms will increase and
menstrual cramping tend to decrease when there is no
ovulation.

Women's bodies produce and have circulating hormones other than estrogen and progesterone that affect their
sexuality. These chemicals are produced and released by
the two adrenal glands located on top of the kidneys. Some
of these hormones are feminizing and some masculizing

(androidal). The ovaries also produce small quantities of androidal hormones. The effects of the feminine and masculine hormones are usually kept in balance except in rare disease states.

During a woman's reproductive years, estrogen overpowers the masculizing effect of the adrenal hormones. But the adrenal glands remain active after menopause. When a woman's ovaries become inactive after menopause and the ovaries no longer release estrogen or progesterone, the adrenal gland hormones can change her sexuality. If the androidal hormones are predominant, facial hair may appear or increase, the clitoris enlarges, the skin produces more oil resulting in acne, and there is usually an increase in libido. More often, there is a close balance between the feminizing and masculizing adrenal hormones, so there is little or no effect on physical or sexual characteristics. However, estrogen deficiency alone can severely affect a woman's personality and sexuality.

Jack Nabors, fifty-eight, arrived at my office with his daughter who was home for the holidays. She and her dad had been talking about his wife, Susan. The daughter had been shocked when she arrived. Her mother appeared to have aged and "seemed different" since her last visit the Christmas before. The daughter was most concerned about her mother's apparent aging. Her posture was slightly stooped over and she looked tired. She also became aware that her mother was extremely moody and behaved differently. When she asked her mother about her health, she was told, rather abruptly, "I'll be fine after I get over these hot flashes."

Jack picked up on this and agreed that his wife did occasionally mention hot flashes and night sweats. He also agreed with his daughter's description of personality changes. Susan had become more sedentary and seemed tired most of the time. He added, "It seems I'm unable to cheer her up like I used to when she became annoyed." He reported that their relationship was now often strained.

I retrieved Susan's medical records and noted she had not been in for two years and had missed her annual health assessment. Her daughter feared her mother might have developed a serious condition such as diabetes or cancer. She asked if I would call Susan and remind her that she was overdue for her physical examination.

The next day Jack called to add to the history he and his daughter had presented at the office. He told me that he had not wanted to say too much in his daughter's presence, but things were even worse than he had described. Susan had become difficult to live with and often became angry over little things. He added, "Frankly, I don't know how much longer I can take it. Her behavior is starting to make me cranky too." Suspecting that Susan might be in a clinical depression, I asked a few more questions including one about their sexual relationship. "There just isn't any," Jack told me. Several months earlier Susan started having some discomfort during intromission and not long after that started, Jack would sometimes lose his erection during coitus. "So we just stopped having intercourse, but that's okay. I guess at my age I shouldn't need sex anymore."

I asked my secretary to call Susan and arrange an appointment. When we met, Susan added several pertinent symptoms to those mentioned by her family. The most troublesome were insomnia and low energy level. But she was also having headaches and her finger joints were stiff in the morning. She attributed the pain during intercourse to vaginal dryness. From the full history I determined that Susan was experiencing menopause and had an estrogen deficiency. I felt but there might be an element of depression as well. Estrogen was started on a diagnostic and therapeutic trial dose, and I made an appointment for her to return in two weeks. I talked to Susan about the various aspects of menopause and its treatment and gave her some reading material and a video tape on the subject.

Susan's return visit was one of those rare and wonderful experiences for a physician—"a therapeutic triumph." She looked like a different woman—her posture had improved, she was carefully groomed, and her happiness was apparent. She told me, "All of those miserable symptoms I had are gone." She ticked them off: insomnia, night sweats, hot flashes, finger stiffness, and headaches. Her energy was restored and she was on a health kick, exercising, and following a better diet.

It was obvious that estrogen deficiency was her only problem. No depression. A few weeks later her husband, Jack sent me a card telling me I was a "miracle worker." I wish treatment for all illnesses could be as successful.

The absence of estrogen in menopausal women causes several physical and psychological changes. The most common are dry vagina during coitus, hot flashes, bladder symptoms such as recurring infections, frequent urination, and urinary discomfort, insomnia, anxiety, irritability, depression, lassitude, and low energy levels. Sexuality typically decreases, but it is not understood whether this is a direct effect of lowered estrogen levels or a psychological response to the other symptoms. However, as mentioned earlier, the hormones released by the adrenal glands and some other psychological factors often compensate for the estrogen decrease and can actually lead to an overall increase in a woman's sexuality after menopause.

How Menopause Affects Men

As a man experiencing male menopause becomes aware of his own decreased libido occurring at the same time that his wife's libido is increasing, he may become distressed. The inability to respond to his wife's sexual wishes or needs can precipitate or worsen his andropausal symptoms. Some men fear that their wives will seek lovers to satisfy their increased sexual needs.

Unfortunately, men often believe that their masculinity is measured by their ability and skill to sexually satisfy women on demand. Any physical manifestation of sexual inadequacy accompanied by fears of further deterioration can be devastating to the man experiencing male menopause. Fortunately, there are solutions to the problem.

The disparity of libido is only a problem for couples who do not communicate their sexual needs and feelings to each other. In a loving relationship, partners are willing to modify their sexual desires somewhat to correlate with those of their spouse, either delaying sexual gratification, or participating in other, non-coital sexual activity if their libido is low. The key to a mutually satisfactory compromise is communication. An additional solution is masturbation in the presence of, or even with the assistance of, the spouse. Sometimes watching a partner masturbate can provide sufficient stimulation to arouse the inactive partner.

Since a man's wife enters menopause around the same time that he enters andropause and since more is known medically about female menopause than about male menopause, learning about the similarities and differences between the two conditions may help him to reach a better understanding of his own symptoms. He may also realize that his menopausal wife's symptoms can directly impact the anxieties and concerns that are part of his viropausal/andropausal condition.

CHAPTER 8

Mature Sex and Love

In mid-life, male sexuality does change, but it does not necessarily diminish (see Chapter 3). Most commonly, men forty-five to sixty need greater, longer, and more various stimulation than they do in their younger years to get an erection and to achieve orgasm. These changes are likely to be perceived as a threat to the andropausal man's masculinity. If he has additional concerns about the possibility of future sexual decline, these can further inhibit his sexuality. If a man's self-image is associated with being a "stud" or a great lover, he may find the mid-life changes in his sexuality especially devastating.

Chapter 6 explored some of the steps a man can take to prevent or reduce his menopausal symptoms, including updating an unrealistically youthful self-image and reordering priorities. Re-examining his sexual self-image and aligning it with physiological reality is another important part of the treatment of male menopause. A middle-aged man who still mentally carries the sexual image of his twenty-year-old self is headed for trouble.

CHAPTER 8

Sexual Self-Image and the Viropause/ Andropause Syndrome

Men seldom discuss changes in sexuality with their friends or even with their doctors, and there's not much literature available, so most men lack both information and appropriate role models who might help them know what to expect sexually in mid-life and how to adjust. As men become better informed, they will realize that their sexuality does not diminish at this time in their lives and that desexualization does not occur. The various aspects of sex, (including but not limited to sexual intercourse) can become, for many reasons, even better and more enjoyable as men drop the compulsion to play a stereotypical macho role. And there is no doubt that their skill at lovemaking can increase with experience. Men who feel free to express their sensitivity and imagination can develop stronger and deeper feelings of total satisfaction and pleasure from sex. They can become innovators and find new ways to express their appreciation of their partner's sexuality and new ways to enjoy sexual activities.

With andropause, men usually think that any change in their sexuality indicates a decrease, and they may seek inappropriate remedies such as affairs with younger, more sexually provocative women. These are only ineffectual band-aid solutions to deeper problems. An effective, permanent solution is to redefine their sexual self-image and to work with their wife or regular sex partner to transform sexual intercourse into a form of gratifying, mature lovemaking.

One of my patients, Carl Sawyer, who was forty-eight, was having problems with his sexual self-image and made an appointment for treatment of his "depression." At his first visit, he did indeed appear depressed. But while I was taking his history, it became apparent that he was not clinically depressed but unhappy. He was hoping that there was some physical explanation for his feeling of dejection. After the examination which show no abnormal physical conditions, he wryly commented, "I guess it's all in my head."

I asked him if he was having any problems at work or at home. "Oh, everything at work is okay, but things could be better at home." With an obvious sense of relief, he described the sequence of changes in his personal life during the previous two years.

A few years previously, Carl felt his life had grown tedious and less interesting. Things at home had developed a routine pattern. He was upset by his apparent reduced sexuality—his wife just didn't excite him as much as she used to—and he was annoyed at the first mild evidence of physical aging. In his restlessness, he had fallen into a sexual affair with Cassie, a young client who was having marital problems and was separated from her husband. Carl was attracted to her youthfulness and physical attributes. Her presence dispelled his feelings of loneliness and unhappiness. He kept telling himself he had a good marriage and it "would be crazy to mess it up" by getting caught in a clandestine affair, but deep down he felt a warm glow and said he hadn't had so much fun since he was in his twenties.

A man experiencing male menopausal symptoms is unable to think clearly. Chaotic emotions and fears distort his thinking about his sexuality. This results in defective ideas, poor planning, and bad decisions. He misinterprets a sexual romance with a younger woman as true love. He considers the temporary increase in his feelings of affection and sexual response to be "normal" and his feelings for his wife suffer by comparison.

Carl started to feel guilty when trying to demonstrate physical affection for his wife. Eventually, she began asking questions about his time away from home and his apparent attitude changes. He hated lying to her. His behavior went against his principles and he lost some of his self-respect, but he refused to see a marriage counselor with her because he knew his relationship with Cassie would be exposed.

After a few more months of trying to live a double life, "all hell broke loose." His wife and he had a serious argument and she accused him of being physically or mentally ill because of his strange behavior and attitude changes. Carl acknowledged the changes to himself but wouldn't admit them to his wife. At the end of the two-hour confrontation she gave him an ultimatum: "Either get help or get out!" In his anger, he packed some clothes and went to a motel.

The man experiencing andropause is supersensitive to criticism. Carl angered quickly and to an extreme level, but his response was mostly due to his feelings of guilt. His anger prevented him from using good judgment, and it seemed easier to move out than to confront the real issues.

Eventually, both Carl and Cassie divorced their spouses and married each other. Since Carl's new marriage was motivated by a short-term increase in his sexuality, anger, and guilt, the new marriage did not go smoothly. There was a lot of tension and animosity between him and Cassie. In his own mind, he had started blaming her for the breakup of his first marriage and was now suffering a great deal of unhappiness and remorse over the whole series of events.

Naturally, I could not undo the events of the past two years for Carl, but I did suggest ways he could self-treat his menopausal syndrome, including adjustments he might make in his attitudes toward his sexuality with his new wife.

During a man's forties and fifties, decreases in a man's sexuality are often related to physical causes such as an illness or excessive drinking, but there are also many possible psychological reasons for mid-life sexual impairment: concern that sexual inadequacy is responsible for the collapse of an affair, guilt produced by cheating on a wife, fear of having acquired a sexually transmitted disease during an extramarital encounter, discomfort during intimacy with a new partner after the death of a wife, criticism from children or friends for remarrying, or feelings of sexual inadequacy after seeing a porno movie.

Carl's reduced sex drive occurred in reaction to the perceived tedium of his home life. If Carl had had access to information about the early symptoms and causes of male menopause, he could have diagnosed himself and learned how to manage the syndrome in its early stages. Or he may have elected to seek professional help.

In the early process of reassessment, Carl might have given more careful thought to his relationship with his wife and why it seemed tedious. "Is it my fault lovemaking has become routine? Do I let her know I truly love her? Am I responsive to loving gestures? Could I make myself more physically appealing?" The biggest question would be "Do I love my wife?" If he answered yes, he would know any amount of effort to improve the relationship was well worth it.

When sexuality is waning, communication with one's

partner is fundamental. The man concerned about his sexuality should let his wife know that he is unhappy with their sex life, being careful not to incriminate her. They should explore the possibilities for improvement together.

He and she might talk about trying something different: a different room, the floor, a new bed, new positions for sexual intercourse—anything but the usual—and including the bizarre and funny, beverages, foods, candles, music, different lighting. . . . Sexual experimentation does wonders for waning libidos.

Often the most effective way couples can renew their sexuality is to take a holiday away together—not a tour or a casino, but somewhere romantic and relaxing like the shore or the mountains, a vacation that will provide unburdened time for talking and exploring. When there is no exhaustion or feeling of animosity, sex takes on new dimensions. Good memories of relaxed sex are carried home and often serve to improve later sexual encounters.

If a man between forty and sixty believes he has a sexuality problem, he should first determine whether or not he is experiencing male menopause. If he can determine this by reading and insight, he may progress on to the next step. If he's unable to make this determination or feels unsure of his diagnosis, he should seek professional advice.

There are many possible explanations for a man's negative sexual self-concept. It can begin during infancy or result from sexual abuse. The teenager is extremely vulnerable to destructive comments and teasing from peers regarding his anatomy as displayed in shower rooms, and a memorable put-down by a date can leave a permanent scar. An insensitive wife may directly or indirectly damage her husband's sexual self-image. Negative self-images can last a lifetime and can exacerbate male menopause, though they don't usually cause it.

When a man in viropause/andropause finds decreasing sexuality is one of his symptoms, each element of the condition must be addressed to achieve a recovery. If only the dwindling sexuality is treated and the other causes left in place, the sexuality problem will probably resurface.

Commonly, the unhappiness (dysphoria) of male menopause prevents normal sexual functioning (libido, erection, and orgasm). Until a man can return to a happy state of mind, free of anxiety, sex will remain a problem. Of course, impaired sexuality can also be one of the causes of male menopause and then should be treated along with the elimination of the other causes such as fear, goal failure, or obsession with aging changes.

If sexual dysfunction is the only reason for a man's andropausal condition, which is rare, a man needs professional attention from a primary physician, urologist, psychiatrist, or sex therapist.

Emotions and Sexual Maturity

During the teens and twenties, there is considerable difference between men and women and their ideas about sex. Although much has changed in male–female physical relationships in the last few decades, it is still the case that many women tend to want a close relationship and affectionate feeling for their partner before they allow themselves to have sex. Men, on the other hand, need only feel a physical attraction to a woman to desire sex with her. In general, young women see sex as a means of expressing their feelings of affection and caring while young men see sex as a means of expressing their maleness and physicality. Following sexual intercourse, women usually feel closer to their partners, but a young man typically loses interest in the woman until the next time he feels a need for sexual gratification.

Observations about young men and women's differences in sexual feelings are not a revelation, but they do serve to remind us of the contrasts between mature sexual feelings and youthful ones. Many women's attitudes and feelings regarding sex mature much earlier than do men's. For many men it is not until they mature and enter into a compatible relationship with their partner that they eventually will include love as a component of sexual intercourse. The realization that a man's feelings of love are connected with physical sex may come to him abruptly, as a revelation, or so gradually that he never really is aware of the change.

Although *making love* is a commonly used term, few of us ever stop to think about what it means. It's often used interchangeably with *coitus* or *sexual intercourse*. In our daily lives we speak very freely about sexual matters, but we are not very sensitive about the real implications or meaning of sex in our lives.

There is a normal and natural evolution that occurs in the relationships of couples who truly love each other. One of the fundamental and extremely important components of the relationship is sex. The pure physical need of youth is supplemented by a spiritual satisfaction as a man falls more deeply in love with his partner. With increasing sexual maturity, sexual intercourse becomes less an act of physical competence and more an act of meaningful love. The transition occurs more quickly when lovers communicate well. As a man becomes aware of these changes he no longer thinks of himself as a great sex machine but rather as a great lover. He realizes that intercourse is an act of love, not a physical feat.

For the man experiencing male menopause this transition doesn't occur; if it does it's delayed. For him this prolonged journey is a series of disappointments and self-degradation.

Sex to most teenage males is strictly a physical experience. To a sexually mature man sex is an aspect of love and appreciation that brings a closeness no other activity can match. The sex act is a statement of past love and a promise of future love for a woman; it invites the ultimate joy of giving and receiving in addition to the extreme pleasure of the physical experience.

The passage from physical sex to mature love is long but rewarding. Of all the things we learn in life, how to become a good lover is the most pleasant. This certainly doesn't imply the knowledge and skill are acquired automatically. After every sexual encounter a man might want to think of what he did right and what he did wrong, how he might improve the experience for himself and for his partner the next time.

Every day we are deluged with what to think about sex, how to feel about sex, and how to perform sex, and, worst of all, we're given standards for sexual performance. The graphic portrayal of physical sex is a big seller and an underlying cause for the unbalanced views we internalize. Is it any wonder some of us today feel underprivileged, unloved, passive, or inadequate if we're not actively practicing frequent, polygamous, kinky sex? Normal, healthy men will recognize this portrayed world of sex as artificial and not feel inadequate if their sexual life does not measure up.

However, andropausal men develop doubts about their own sexuality when exposed to these inputs.

Developing true sexual maturity is a natural process. A man learns through observing his own sexual experiences, evaluating these experiences, and then using what he learns in the process. Like many things learned in life, trial and error play an important role. Different approaches to sex, different sexual communication, and different techniques can bring greater satisfaction.

When the sexual maturing process moves towards less concern for self and more concern for a partner, a man will find more and more satisfaction. As his ability to show affection and deep caring grows, so does his ability to enjoy a rich, full sexual relationship. He is rewarded richly by his partner showing the same feeling toward him. As he matures, the physical aspects of coitus becomes less important than the emotional and loving aspects. This is not to say he doesn't want and need physical gratification.

Lest the mature sex sounds quieter and less robust, certain aspects of the physical, mature love must be emphasized. The sounds of pleasure, vigorous movements, heavy breathing, and sex talk are part of mature sex as much as they are of purely physical sexual activity. The moans, groans, and shrieks may be as loud and frequent. The experimentation in position may be as varied. Innovative modification, such as the use of a vibrator, are as common. Stimuli such as books and movies are still used. Mature sex has all the wonderful benefits of physical sex plus the very important feelings of love and true intimacy.

Communicating About Sex and Love

Love can survive and grow without sex, but for most of

us, sex is an extremely important factor in our primary loving relationship.

Various forms of the physical expression of love, especially intercourse, are wonderful and strong ways of saying, "I love you." When two mature people love each other, they naturally try to please each other. But, contrary to what many of us think, good sexual experiences do not just happen for a couple. Most of us do intuit, consciously or unconsciously, what feels good to and satisfies our partner and this intuition then becomes part of our behavior in subsequent lovemaking. Intuitive responding and relating usually works well, up to a point, but it may not be enough. Sometimes a partner's sexual signals are misread; but even if they're not, good sex can be made better. To achieve that improvement, couples need to talk to each other about how and what they are feeling.

Most partners say, "I love you" or words to that effect while having intercourse. Other verbalized sounds, including moans, groans, and screams while climaxing also tell a partner that he or she is much loved, as do the physical acts which evoke them. These forms of communication are important, but partners can increase their intimacy and pleasure even further by talking to each other about what they like or dislike all though the sexual act.

The form that communication about sex takes varies for any couple. During the physical expression of love it may consist of only a few words: "Does this feel good?" "Put your hand a little lower." "Don't press quite so hard." "I like it when you do that." "I come quicker when you do this." "I like to feel your smooth, soft skin here." Positive statements and suggestions are easier to accept and respond to than negative statements or criticisms. The communication can also include an interchange of a few sentences during the arousal phase or after orgasm and withdrawal. The petting (arousal) and post-coital stages offer non-threatening times for talking about sex. Inhibitions are lowest after sex and talking at this time increases the feelings of closeness and relaxation. Talking before sex increases the feeling of intimacy and heightens anticipation; it heightens the meaning of the experience.

Some topics of sexual talk may be intimate and very physical: "Do you like strong, fast thrusting as you near orgasm, or do you like more deliberate thrusting?" "I like it when you put your hands on my buttocks while I'm coming; where do you like my hands?" Other topics may not be as intimate but can still help improve the sexual activity. "Do you mind when I forget to shave before coming to bed?" "I like soft music on while we're making love." "Let's make love here on the floor in front of the fire tonight." "The fragrance of your old after shave lotion turned me on more than this new one does." "It seems we both express stronger sexual feelings when the children are out of the house."

Longer discussions may be appropriate if a couple is developing problems in their physical relationship. As long as there is mutual love and a positive attitude, talking can often resolve problems. Subjects for discussion might include the time of day that is most suitable for lovemaking, the preferred physical surroundings, the level of privacy, the amount of light, the temperature, the acceptability of planned or spontaneous demonstrations of love, acceptability of coitus during the menstrual period, acceptable and desirable positions during intercourse, acceptability of oral sex, and a partner's hygiene habits. Asking a partner about what he or she wants is a sign of love and caring.

Selecting an appropriate time and circumstances for talking about lovemaking is of utmost importance. Naturally, both partners should feel like talking about sex for the conversation to be productive. Generally, the talks will go better at a time when both partners are rested and feel free of stress. When a person is tired or focused on some other concern, he or she will probably not be receptive to suggestions and might perceive them as criticism.

Cocktail hour, before dinner can be a good time to discuss important subjects. Whether this is a productive choice depends on the couple and whether there are children or others present. If one feels physically or mentally fatigued because of the day's demands, touchy subjects should be avoided. However, if there is a feeling of relief and of having left behind the pressures of the day and a couple is alone, it can be a good time. A drink or two can have a relaxing effect and help the couple to be more receptive and imaginative. However, excessive drinking dulls the senses and can turn moods in a negative direction.

Couples should choose a time for their discussion when outside distractions are likely to be minimal. Loud music in a nearby room, interruptions from the kids, or a ringing telephone, for example, can cut off or inhibit a free discussion.

Vacations or holidays when the couple is alone together are excellent times to discuss sex. The atmosphere, relaxation, and closeness of these times are conducive to good conversation. The ride home after a happy holiday experience comes close to the ideal time and circumstance for talking, unless the holiday has been exhausting or there are troubling thoughts about what is expected at home or at work. Couples with children may have to work at creating times when they can be alone and when they are not too exhausted to talk. Maintaining a good relationship should include scheduling time for such verbal intimacy.

It is helpful to establish ground rules in advance for talks regarding sex. For example, discussions when there are feelings of anger or resentment are destructive. Sex is a delicate topic for most people, and discussions should stop when either partner feels angry. It is best to briefly explain any bad feelings and ask to discuss the matter at another time. However, the discussion should not be postponed too long, because the problems will not go away simply because they are not discussed.

If elements of the discussion seem distasteful to either partner, the one who is offended should say so and ask to redirect the conversation so it is not offensive. That does not mean that sensitive subjects should not be discussed, but only that couples should be aware of each other's sensibilities and discuss their concerns in terms that do not offend the other.

During her annual gynecological examination, a patient of mine, Barbara Howard, forty-six, recounted several areas of disagreement with her husband. She said they were very upsetting to her and complained about her husband's unwillingness to discuss differences. "He goes into another room and sometimes even goes to his office downtown." She was experiencing increasing anxiety that seemed to be related to friction between her and her husband. Early in the conversation she assured me, "I love my husband as much as I ever did, and that's probably why our fighting bothers me so much." Over the preceding years I considered theirs a good, solid marriage. Hoping to salvage it I suggested another appointment to talk more about the stress she was experiencing. She very willingly agreed.

During our next consultation, Barbara's descriptions of her arguments with her husband spilled out more rapidly and were punctuated by gentle weeping and wiping of her eyes. Near the end of the hour she admitted what was really worrying her: "I'm scared to death he's interested in someone else and that he'll want a divorce." I asked her if she thought her husband would come to our next consultation. She responded, "He probably won't want to, but I'll give it a try."

A week later I was pleasantly surprised when they both arrived for her appointment. Barbara's husband, Jim, appeared a little embarrassed but seemed cooperative. I encouraged them both to talk about the problems they were experiencing. The conversation flowed quite smoothly, but it was obvious there were unresolved problems between them with some of hostility surfacing from time to time. To my question to each of them, "Do you love him/her?" they both responded with a strong yes. "So, you want marriage counseling, not divorce counseling," I said with a smile. When I asked about their sexual relationship they both looked uncomfortable, but agreed, "Our sex life is okay." However, Jim called the next day to tell me that sex was actually one of their biggest problems. "She's never liked sex very much, but it's gotten worse." I suggested they make an appointment to discuss this aspect of the relationship. He agreed and a time was set.

Jim arrived without Barbara. He explained that she didn't think sex was a cause of their misunderstandings and she told him he could go by himself if he wanted. He started the conversation by saying, "As you know, my wife was brought up in a very religious family and talk of sex was taboo." Barbara had lived a sheltered life both at home and at school. Her parents had been overprotective and limited her exposure to the outside world—they closely monitored and restricted such things as books and movies. Her high school education was in a church school and she attended a church-operated college in a neighboring state where she met her husband. His home life and schooling were similar to hers and neither had dated much. After they met, the relationship developed rapidly and they married at the end of their second year of college.

Jim went on to describe their sexual relationship. Barbara had never had an orgasm. She told him early in their marriage she loved him very much but did not need sex as part of her love and that she would be "willing to have sex" when he needed it. Beyond that they talked very little about sexual matters. Their routine was to have intercourse once weekly on Saturday night.

With three children in college and only the youngest at home, their interests diverged, and the relationship—including their sexual relationship—deteriorated. Jim had become successful and had fewer worries and concerns about his business, so his mind was free to think of other things. One of these things was sex. He began reading novels that had graphic sexual scenes. It was then he began seeing women through different eyes. He realized he needed and wanted more from their weekly sexual encounters. During the previous two years he had suggested to Barbara that they vary their sex activity, including the timing.

He also suggested his wife read some of the novels. After reading half of the first novel Barbara told him she didn't care for the book and "found parts of it disgusting."

When this approach didn't work, Jim took a more direct approach. When he became more aggressive, she indicated surprise and said things such as, "What are you doing? You spend too much time reading those books." She met his amorous advances with a coldness that left him feeling embarrassed and resentful. She also rejected any sexual experimentation. After several weeks of being rejected he gave up and returned to the old routine. However, he found himself thinking more and more about sex and embarrassingly admitted he found himself looking at some of his female employees and mentally visualizing them with their clothes off. He soon started experiencing occasional erection failures. It was then that his wife became alarmed and began worrying about their relationship, as indicated during the gynecological exam.

Both Barbara and Jim came to the next consultation. I did not bring up the subject of sex but spent most of the time talking to them about the need for marital counseling. They were both reluctant and indicated that they would not feel comfortable talking about their troubles with a stranger, but they finally agreed when I pointed out their love for each other was too valuable and important to lose. I was careful to suggest counselors who were qualified to give sex guidance.

A month later I received a consultation report from the therapist they had selected. She indicated the couple's major problem was their sexual differences, but she was certain they would be able to solve their problem. After another three months she reported the regular visits were terminated because the couple had made rapid progress.

The following year during Barbara's gynecological exam, she reported to me that things were much better since she had rid herself of her "old-fashioned ideas about sex." She added, with no embarrassment, that she didn't know sex could be so good and was sorry she'd missed so much in her first twenty-two years of marriage.

The therapist was successful in getting Barbara to change her inhibited attitudes about sex. Under her guidance, Barbara and her husband developed much better communication in various areas of their relationship including sex. This opened up a whole new world to both. Their sexual encounters were more frequent and often spontaneous. They had started camping and cross-country skiing together and had re-established a loving relationship. Now, when camping, they sought isolated locations so they could make love outdoors. After these encounters they talked more about intimate subjects as well as new interests they shared.

If either partner believes a couple's sexual or relational problems are not resolvable by mutual discussion, it is advisable for the couple to seek counseling. It is well to remember that if one member of a couple has a problem, both have a problem. In a relationship, neither partner can act unilaterally about sexual matters and neither can dictate how the other feels or should feel. If sincere discussion doesn't resolve the problem or improve the couple's feelings about the issue, expert help is needed. However, before concluding that sex counseling is appropriate, several conversations are needed, with time in between for both partners to think about what's been said. Sex counseling can be very effective provided that each partner loves the other, cares about what the other wants, and truly desires to improve their sex life together.

There are some nonverbal signals that let us know when sexual communications need improvement: When sexual activity becomes ritualized or less spontaneous it may be time to talk sex; if either partner finds acquaintances more interesting than before, especially if either becomes more flirtatious, a bit of lighthearted but meaningful talking might forestall future problems. If sleep regularly takes precedence over love making it might be that tiredness is not the real reason. Talk about it.

We all have had childhood sex experiences. Most of them are innocent and have little bearing on our adult sexuality, so the memories can be shared without much embarrassment and can serve as an introduction to future discussions about sex. How, as children, we may have responded to accidentally seeing adult sexual activity, to seeing animals copulate, or our early ideas about where babies came from are amusing and non-threatening subjects that can serve to move the conversation to the more sensitive but important subject of how and what formed our feelings and ideas about sex. Religious and secular training from parents and gossip from school friends have profound effects on our adult sexual standards, thinking, and behavior. Sharing these memories with each other is of tremendous benefit in understanding our own and our partner's sexual beliefs and responses.

Probably the most touchy subject involves revealing details of previous adult experiences. For some couples, this topic can be a source of closeness, but for others it can leave permanent wounds. There are probably no good rules for handling this subject, so it should be approached slowly and very carefully. Finally the discussion should move to talking about the here and now of the current sexual relationship

Inasmuch as a powerful and frequent cause of male

menopause is inadequate communication, the communication channel for sexual matters must be kept open to prevent the condition. If the channel closes a man is at high risk of becoming andropausal.

Sex is the spice of love. A meal may be nutritious without spice, but the spice elevates a meal to a gourmet delight. The most wondrous and enduring experience is to love and be loved. Sex can and should be more than a ritual to satisfy a physical need. Communication helps the beauty of sex enrich any loving relationship.

CHAPTER 9

Sexual Dysfunction

Most of the current medical and media interest in male menopause focuses on the fears and realities of men's mid-life loss of virility: the lessening of the sex drive, less firmness of the penis, impotence, and delayed orgasm. These are probably the most visible and dramatic symptoms and tend to produce the most anxiety in men experiencing the viropause/andropause syndrome. However, though these elements certainly play an important role among the causes of male menopause, they are not male menopause itself. Physical sexual dysfunction may precede or intensify viropause/andropause, but it is not the sole or even most important cause of the syndrome.

As we discussed in Chapter 3, many of the symptoms of sexual dysfunction men fear actually reflect the small, natural changes that commonly occur in mid-life sexuality and are not in any way to be considered as dysfunctional. If there is a physical problem of a sexual nature such as consistent (rather than occasional) impotency or total inability to achieve orgasm, these problems must be treated as would any other medical conditions such as indigestion, joint stiffness, or back aches.

Nicholas Vining looked very unhappy. He was fifty-one and he and his were had recently separated when he first visited my office. His chief complaint was erectile failure. The problem had first appeared nine months earlier as an occasional problem and had progressed rapidly over the next eight weeks. When I saw him, he hadn't had an erection in seven months.

The laboratory tests we conducted established a diagnosis of diabetes. According to his history, the disease had been present for at least four years. When we discussed his problem he recalled having had an insurance examination required by his employers at which he had been told he had "sugar in his urine" and was advised to see his physician. However, since he had no symptoms he had disregarded the advice.

It is not unusual for incipient adult diabetes to escalate in the viropausal/andropausal years. In addition to having diabetes, Nick was twenty-four percent over his ideal weight and was drinking a six-pack of beer daily. Additional laboratory studies indicated reduced blood flow to the penis. I also noted that due to both personal and physical problems, Nick exhibited an unhappy state of mind and confusion about his goals for the future.

I explained to him that uncontrolled diabetics develop significant artery disease at an earlier age than nondiabetics, and it progresses rapidly. Unfortunately the condition is irreversible. I hastened to discuss possible solutions, such as penile prostheses, vacuum devices, and the possibility of penile injections. I gave him literature and audio cassettes to help him in his decision.

I also explained the other symptoms of male menopause that he seemed to be exhibiting and told him these too could be eliminated through counseling and self-examination.

In the months that followed, Nick chose on of the methods I had suggested of solving his diabetes-induced impotence, and together we explored solutions to his other andropausal problems.

There are many physical components of male menopause, but the basic and most important elements of the syndrome are psychological and behavioral. To be successful, any treatment of male menopause, whether self-directed or professional, must address the total syndrome, not just the physical or sexual aspects.

Kevin Lowry was a new patient when he arrived in my office "to have a cholesterol check." Kevin was fifty-six. He had made the appointment a few days after his older brother, age fifty-nine, had suffered a heart attack. There was additional family history of heart attacks. Kevin's grandfather had his first myocardial infarction at age sixty-two and died with the second attack at age sixty-six. His father developed angina at fifty-seven and a year later had surgery for a coronary bypass.

Like most adults, Kevin knew something of the relationship between blood cholesterol and heart disease. He appeared rather tense, so I spent a little time talking to him of general things, hoping to make him more comfortable. I obtained a general history, performed a physical examination, and ordered blood tests and an electrocardiogram. I was very much relieved when the examination and tests were essentially normal, including the lipid screen (cholesterol, triglycerides, HDL, and LDL). It appeared Kevin had inherited his mother's genes.

As I continued to make notes on his history, unrelated but important symptoms emerged. For four years Kevin had been experiencing fatigue and lassitude. He was having headaches, indigestion, nighttime urination, and discomfort in both knees. Personal history revealed a high coffee and alcohol intake. His noon meals with friends were usually hamburgers preceded by two martinis. He prepared his own inadequate evening meal, but more often he went to a restaurant. After others had left the office he drank two double scotches while clearing his desk of the papers that had accumulated through the day. This was followed by more scotch at home and a half a bottle of red wine with the evening meal. He also smoked a pack of cigarettes a day.

Kevin told me he was a weekend athlete. He had been a "physical person" all his life following sports in high school and college. His weekends were filled with tennis, skiing, and running, plus weight lifting when he had the time. On Mondays and Tuesdays he had to use ibuprofen to relieve the pain in his knees from his weekend sports activities.

Kevin was already achieving success as a financial adviser when he married at the age of thirty-four. When he was forty-five, he fell into an affair with a younger woman. His marriage fell apart, and after thirteen years of marriage and no children, he and his wife were divorced. Soon thereafter the affair cooled and he began a series of sexual relationships as brief as one night and never longer than eight months.

When Kevin was about fifty-three he became aware of

some subtle changes in his body. He started balding, his waist expanded, and he needed glasses for reading. He also noticed that it took him longer to recover from physical activities. He didn't want to let the years change him or his lifestyle, so he signed up for a fitness course, replaced his wardrobe with more youthful clothes, and started dating younger women. He swallowed a handful of vitamin, mineral, and protein supplements every day.

About the same time he discovered he was finding less pleasure in life. His work seemed less challenging and more monotonous. Some of his associates were taking early retirement. This jolted him. Maybe soon he would be retiring and his income from work would drop off.

In addition, he didn't find his new sex partners sufficiently stimulating and he started noticing a reduction in his sexuality. His sex drive was sporadic and his erections were sometimes delayed in spite of more unusual and vigorous stimulation. On one occasion, after a long and exhausting thrusting effort, he wasn't able to reach orgasm. The frustration of this failure preyed on his mind for days. "I'm really losing it."

By the time he came to my office he had strong feelings of "sliding down the slippery slope." His brother's heart attack precipitated fear and anxiety about his own mortality. Until then he had been successful in pushing the thoughts of life's terminating into the subconscious.

Kevin was greatly relieved to learn that his lipids were okay. However, he was obviously distressed when I spoke of other heart risk factors, all of which were as important as the lipids. We talked of his excessive alcohol intake. I encouraged him to limit the intake to no more than two drinks a day and, most important, to totally discontinue cigarette smoking. We also discussed his selecting more appropriate exercise.

I discovered that Kevin had a typical case of andropause. During his office visits I gradually introduced him to the concept. He was able to recognize how his fears about his health and sexuality fit the pattern.

Most men suffering from male menopause do have some degree of sexual impairment or at least have concerns about their sexuality. If the sexual impairment is due to a physical condition, it should be treated both for itself and because sexual dysfunction can cause or intensify male menopause.

Physical Causes of Sexual Dysfunction
Diabetes

Diabetes is a common physical cause of sexual impairment in men. This chronic disease eventually reduces blood supply to organs of the body, including heart, eyes, brain, and genitalia. Penile erection occurs when more blood flows into the penis than flows out so an imbalance in blood circulation will negatively affect the normal response of the penis to erotic stimulation. Many people are aware of diabetes and how it relates to other symptoms, but few know that the inability to get an erection may be one of its earliest observable signs. Unfortunately, if diabetes has progressed to this point, the impotence is often irreversible. Men who come from families with a history of adult-type diabetes should be tested for diabetes regularly whether or not there are any symptoms. Diabetes can be diagnosed from a simple blood sugar test that can be done as a regular feature of the annual physical at the doctor's office.

Hypertension

Hypertension, or elevated blood pressure, does not impair sexual function. However, one of its complications, artery disease, does in its more advanced stages. Unfortunately, many of the medications administered to control high blood pressure interfere with sexuality. Some also cause a mild depression. Two of the manifestations of depression are reduced sex drive (for women also) and impotence. If either change occurs while taking high blood pressure medication, adjustment in dosage or change to a different medication can reverse the depression and allow the libido to return to normal. Some medications produce a fatigue syndrome, and also interferes with sexual vigor.

Sex after Heart Attacks

For decades myocardial infarcts (heart attacks) were believed to be caused by anxiety. Doctors would tell the family members of the heart patient, "Don't let him get upset; he'll have another heart attack." The myth persists that an emotional upset is the cause of heart attack, although that theory was disproved by medical science many years ago. Heart attack victims and their spouses may, after the diagnosis of a heart attack is established, begin to worry about sex. The worry can increase to near panic: "No more sex!"

Sexual activity in its many forms is an important part of most couples' relationships. There is a physical need to express love through intercourse. It is an intimacy that cannot be ended without injury to the relationship. Very strong reassurance is usually required from their doctor before a couple's fears about sex after a heart attack can be dispelled. The person who suffered the heart attack usually experiences the most fear.

When I am counseling a couple after a heart attack, I know that I have to be direct, precise, and explicit in my discussion. The statement "Oh, sure, you can have sex" is not adequate. Couples want to know a precise date when sex can be resumed and what amount of physical activity is considered appropriate. Resuming sex requires a gradual adjustment just as does the resumption of any other form of physical exercise. Just as a heart attack patient gradually returns to such activities as walking, jogging, and working, so it is with sex.

Most couples have difficulty talking openly about sex, even though it is important to them. However, this is a time they need to ask their doctor for a graphic explanation of such sexual topics as acceptable positions, the vigor of thrusting, whether orgasm should be inhibited, and whether sexual activity should be avoided after meals.

Sometimes men who have suffered a heart attack are afraid to admit that they fear the possibility of having another heart attack as a result of having sex. That fear can be a strong deterrent to open discussion about sex with their doctors or wives. Because male heart attack victims are likely to be unable to even confront that fear, a wife should ask the doctor to explain things that might not otherwise be asked. A man's ego is intimately involved with his sexuality, as well as his concept of courage, so the doctor is confronting a complex psychological issue when he counsels heart attack victims about sex. In addition to deep psychic fears, the patient must also deal with the unfortunate popular myths about heart attacks. In spite of what movies and novels tell us, men do not expire in the act of coitus. A man who recovers from a heart attack can expect to be able to physically express his love without fear. To borrow some words that seem particularly apt, he has nothing to fear but fear itself.

Despite the myths, men recovering from heart attacks are not supposed to refrain from sex or other forms of physical exertion. Doctors often test heart attack victims with treadmill electrocardiograms soon after attacks, and these tests are more strenuous than vigorous sex. Sexual intercourse requires about the same amount of physical exertion as climbing two flights of stairs and should be performed at the same graduated levels of stair climbing by the newly recovering heart attack patient. Heart attacks do not, by any means, end a man's ability to express sexual love.

Chemical Abuse

Drug and alcohol abuse are extremely common causes of sexual dysfunction. Chemical abuse can reduce libido, prevent or end an erection, and prevent or delay orgasm. Both legal (alcohol and prescription drugs) and illegal chemicals are implicated. The chemicals in cigarettes also accelerate artery disease and impair sexual function. As noted by Shakespeare, a small amount of alcohol encourages sexual activity, but more decreases it. A drink or two may reduce inhibitions, but excessive alcohol consumption before intercourse, as well as chronic use, impairs sexual function. Acute alcohol intoxication affects mental concentration, so the intense erotic thought process is interrupted. Intoxication also deters physical function.

Chronic excessive use of alcohol is the most common chemical abuse in sexual dysfunction observed by clinicians in their practices. This is especially noticeable for patients fifty and over. Two ounces of hard liquor per day is usually tolerated well. (One shot of hard liquor, one twelve-ounce beer, and one glass of wine are approximate equivalents.) Some men are less sensitive to the effects of alcohol and experience no impairment even with large amounts. But men who are experiencing any sexual problems are encouraged to abstain from alcohol for one month as a diagnostic and therapeutic measure.

Because sexual performance depends greatly on the thought process, illegal drugs affect libido, potency, and orgasms. The effect is almost totally adverse. As with alcohol, the illegal drug effect on sexuality is related to dose and the individual baseline sexuality. The triggering mechanism for orgasm is in the mind. It requires intense, highly selective thought direction. Drugs impair this function. The sex-suppressing effects are produced by drugs derived from the opium plant (codeine, morphine, heroin), the cocoa plant (cocaine, "crack"), and the mescaline plant (hallucinogens), as well as from some synthesized drugs such as "speed."

There are many myths about the potentiating effects of drugs on sex drive and sexual performance. Cannabis (marijuana) is similar to alcohol in reducing inhibitions in lesser doses, so it has been suggested to act as an aphrodisiac. In reality, larger doses and chronic use can reduce sexuality.

A large number of prescription drugs also affect sexual function, but usually only to a slight degree. The most commonly prescribed drugs that suppress sexual function are high blood pressure medications. There is not complete agreement about this, but many clinicians are reluctant to prescribe or continue the use of these agents for men who have impairment of their sexuality. Fortunately, there are several medications that are effective in high blood pressure treatment, so the physician has the option of choosing one or more which may not display sex suppression.

Tranquilizers in general, depending on dose, decrease libido and responsiveness in some users. The older medications used for anxiety, the barbiturates, have a delaying effect on orgasm. Some men taking Phenobarbital, for instance, are completely incapable of having an orgasm. On the other hand, if a person has extreme anxiety and is incapable of having any interest in sex, an appropriate tranquilizer in proper dosage can be beneficial.

A common symptom of depression is reduced or complete absence of sex drive. The present-day medications for depression are very effective in controlling the condition, thus restoring libido. In a few patients, both men and women, these medications delay or prevent orgasm. This reaction to the medication needs consideration of both the patient and the physician in the selection of which medication to use and to the dosage.

A group of medications classified as anticholenergics affect sexual function in some patients, most notably by delaying orgasm. They are used for gastrointestinal conditions, such as gastritis, peptic ulcers, and irritable bowel syndrome. Many of the over-the-counter antihistamines are chemically and pharmacologically related to the anticholenergics in their effects.

External Causes

Severe illnesses, acute and chronic, often impair sexual function. Men perform best when they are feeling robust and strong. Men who feel poorly often suffer temporarily from low libido or impotence. For example, a man suffering from a case of flu is not usually sexually inclined. Those who are weakened and miserable with chronic or serious illness likewise are less libidinous.

Similarly, those recovering from severe accidents often experience sexuality impairments. However, victims of accidents, after recovery, are not impaired. For example, medical research is replete with cases of vigorous and satisfying sexual activity after loss of a limb and even for those left paraplegic. On the other hand, those surviving severe head injuries may be asexual, depending on the extent and part of the brain that's been damaged. Interestingly, men who have the misfortune of losing both testes often can perform sexually, provided the loss occurs after normal secondary sex organ developments. Research shows the effect of castration on libido is not consistent.

Medical Solutions to Physical Impotence

There are increasing numbers of articles in lay publications suggesting that impotence is commonly caused by physical rather than psychological factors. Often these articles treat the subject superficially. Usually, if the originating scientific data is quoted, it will show the high percentages attributed to physical causes are not for men in their viropausal/andropausal years, but men sixty or older. Actually, the percentage of physically caused impotence is very low, probably accounting for less than five percent of physically normal men. Impotency for physical reasons begin in the sixth decade, and the incidence then is related to age.

There are two medical procedures available for treating impotence. Surgical insertion of penile implants (prostheses) is a satisfactory solution to the problem of physical impotence for many men. There is increasing use of the implant because of recent improvement in both the devices and in the necessary surgical skills. More and more men seek this procedure as they learn of their male acquaintances who have accepted this means of restoring sexual capability. Both patients and their wives are very appreciative (after healing is complete) when the power to express love sexually is restored.

Recently, an external vacuum chamber device has been introduced for the management of erection difficulties. It consists of a clear plastic cylinder and a pumping mechanism. The penis is inserted into the tube and a negative pressure (vacuum) is created around the penis. An erection develops promptly and a plastic ring is placed at the base of the penis to maintain the erection. The device is available with either a hand pump or a battery-operated pump. This external device is gaining popularity among patients; physicians who prescribe them report a high percentage of patients who are satisfied with this method. There have been no major side effects reported. However, the suitability of this device must be determined by a patient's physician, and only prescribed devices obtained through an authorized medical outlet should be used. Men should not attempt self-treatment with similar devices available through mail-order catalogues without a prescription. With mail-order devices, there is a definite possibility of permanent damage.

Because sexual dysfunction is occasionally due to physical abnormalities that are correctable, the patients, with the help of their physicians, should consider these as possible causes and rule them out before proceeding with a psychological approach. Whether the cause is physical or psychological, a proper diagnosis is important so the underlying condition—hormones, metabolism, anxiety, depression, or extrinsic factors—can be properly treated. Diagnosis is also needed to determine if the impotence is related to andropausal factors. Treatments for impotence vary depending on the initial cause; treatment for any one condition will most likely not be the treatment of choice for another.

Psychological Causes of Sexual Dysfunction
Depression

There are several mental conditions that interfere with sexual function such as neuroses (hypochondriacally, obsessive disorder, compulsive disorder, phobia) and psychoses (delusional paranoia, schizophrenia, manic depression). The two most common mental conditions may occur in the absence of male menopause but frequently are associated with it: anxiety and depression.

Depression is now believed to be a "chemical" disturbance in the central nervous system, so perhaps it should not be considered a truly psychological condition. But because it affects thinking and feelings, it is usually thought of as psychological in nature. The more common symptoms of depression are unhappiness, dysphoria (feeling of ill-being, discontent), fatigue, low energy level, withdrawal, altered eating or sleeping patterns, reduced mental acuity, impaired memory, and reduced sexuality.

Contrary to common belief, depression is not a response to bad events. A common response of a man who has been informed that he suffers from depression is "It can't be; I have nothing to be depressed about." Clinical depression usually occurs without external causes.

It has been estimated that depression occurs sometime during the life of over forty million adults in this country.

Depression may vary in severity from feeling mildly disturbed to feeling suicidal. In recent years many antidepressive medications have become available. They work, it is believed, by correcting the "chemical" imbalance at the nerve endings of the brain cells.

Thoughts of sex just don't enter the head of most depressed men. If a man who is severely depressed attempts sexual intercourse, the likely result is failure—erectile or orgasmic failure or both. That failure adds to his depression, and frequently a depressed man develops guilt feelings about being unable to sexually express his love for his partner. This concern can lead to anxiety superimposed on his depression.

The condition of depression is frequently self-limiting. There is often a spontaneous recovery after months or years. But because the illness is prolonged and, to some degree, disabling, treatment is advisable. The best treatment is usually a combination of counseling and medications. Most of the counseling for depression is provided by primary physicians who also prescribe the medications. Psychiatrists, who have M.D.s, can also provide both. The use of medication is almost always successful. In choosing a medication, the physician attempts to select the one most appropriate to the individual's needs.

One drawback of antidepressant medications are occasional mild side effects. These include mouth dryness, constipation, increased appetite, drowsiness, or insomnia. Fortunately, side effects usually subside with longer use and dose adjustment.

Antidepressants are not sedatives or tranquilizers so they do not impair sexual function (except in the case of a few patients who experience delayed orgasm). Because depression reduces sexuality and the medication can delay orgasm, the patient and the physician must work together in selecting the medication and timing of administration, as well as dosage.

Anxiety

Anxiety is a common mental disorder. People use various words and phrases when referring to their feelings that are indications they are suffering from anxiety. They may refer to themselves as being "nervous," "anxious," "apprehensive," "uptight," "stressed," "under tension," or "shaky inside." All of us experience anxiety to some degree every day. When it occurs with real causes—that is, when it is the result of stressors—it is a normal response. When it occurs without an identifiable cause, it is abnormal. In addition, it is abnormal when the degree of response to stressors is unreasonable. There are several different types of anxiety. They include generalized anxiety, adjustment disorder anxiety, social anxiety, various phobias, panic, and agoraphobia. Generalized anxiety is the type that most often results in sexual problems.

Roger Lyle came to see me three weeks after his fifty-eighth birthday about his recent problem with impotence. He had remarried five months before and introduced the subject by saying, "Jane is a wonderful wife, but sometimes I just can't get it up. It's not her fault; she's really sexy."

A physical exam and lab tests ruled out a physical explanation for his impotence. He did not have diabetes, blood vessel disease, or a hormonal deficiency, so I concluded the cause was psychological.

Roger had been divorced from his first wife of twenty-five years just a few years earlier. After their children had left home, he and his wife realized that they had little in common and that their life together, including their sex life, had become ritualistic and boring. The divorce was by mutual agreement and uncontested by either.

Roger and Jane had known each other thirty-five years earlier in college. She had moved away after college, married, and had two children. She returned to her home town after her husband died of a heart attack. After her return, Jane and Roger's old friendship developed into an intimate relationship. They were married when Roger was fifty-seven and Jane fifty-three.

Roger described their early sexual encounters as "highly successful." He described in some detail his erections and orgasms. "My sexual performance was as good as when I was in my twenties." It was about a month before his office visit that he had a sexual failure. It occurred shortly before midnight on a Friday. That had been a stressful day at work, and he felt mentally fatigued. He had two highballs while dressing for a party at the country club, so by the time they arrived at the party he was "feeling no pain." They danced after dinner and he continued to drink until he left the party.

They were both in a happy, loving mood when they arrived home and felt motivated to express their love physically. Roger's erection was quick and of good hardness, but after thrusting for a minute or two, he lost the erection. No amount of effort by his wife or himself returned the firmness. He was frustrated and unable to get to sleep. Jane's reassurances did little to dispel his misery.

He thought about this sexual failure nearly every day when his mind was not otherwise actively engaged. For example, when driving home after work, he would plan the evening with Jane and wonder if he was going to "be a good lover or poop out." Most of the time he was capable of adequate thrusting, but "it was not as good, not the same." Other times he was unable to have an erection or lost it while thrusting.

As I have said before, sexuality begins waning slightly during a man's thirties, but is usually not troublesome until his fifties. Concern about this change is one of the frequent fears that causes the male menopause. For many men, fear of losing their total sexual capability is devastating. Fortunately, the fear can be eliminated and satisfactory sexual functioning restored.

Since Roger's impotence was related to fatigue, alcohol, stress, and the accompanying anxiety—in other words, andropausal and lifestyle factors and not disease of hormonal deficiency—some counseling and information on male menopause was sufficient for his recovery from impotence.

Almost every patient who experiences anxiety can relate his bad feelings to some problem in his life. The most common problems are related to work, personal relationships, and real (or perceived) illness. If the response to the problem is inappropriate, it is considered an illness, and this illness can be destructive to normal sexual function.

Anxiety reduces a man's libido. The thought processes necessary for a healthy sexual appetite are crowded out by disturbing thoughts that fill the mind of the anxious man.

Anxiety also produces mental fatigue, and this type of fatigue is a strong deterrent to sex. Mental fatigue, with or without anxiety, is a very common cause of reduced libido and impotence. On the other hand, physical fatigue, unless extreme, does not impair sexual function.

Anxiety is often treated by the use of sedatives or tranquilizers. While they relieve the feelings of anxiety, they are usually not appropriate in the treatment of sexual problems. It is important to know that, like alcohol, these medications may interfere with the normal mental and physical activity needed for good sexual performance. Moreover, this sometimes has a domino effect—the reduced sexuality can further increase the anxiety—so the man being treated for anxiety needs to discuss the various possibilities with his doctor.

CHAPTER 10

Testosterone Deficiency

On September 28, 1992, the ABC television show "20/20" ran a segment on the hormone testosterone with the implicit assumption that testosterone therapy might be indicated as a general and safe treatment for men experiencing male menopause, just as the corresponding hormone estrogen is prescribed for a large majority of menopausal and post-menopausal women. In my medical opinion this is a dangerous assumption based on unpublished anecdotal material rather than on exacting medical research.

Testosterone is the primary hormone produced by the testes and is under the control of hormones secreted by the pituitary gland. Testosterone is responsible for male secondary characteristics: deep voice, facial and pubic hair growth, larger muscles, and so on. In later life it accelerates baldness. Sufficient testosterone is produced throughout a lifetime well into the nineties, unlike estrogen, which is no longer produced by women after menopause. In the normal, healthy male, testosterone levels start dropping in the sixth decade, while the onset of male menopause is usually in the fourth or fifth decades. The amount of testosterone produced by the normal man starts decreasing gradually in the sixties, but it never drops low enough to interfere significantly with sexuality.

Hormonal deficiencies in middle-aged men, including testosterone deficiency, are seldom a contributing cause of the male menopause syndrome; in fact, very few men under the age of sixty-five suffer at all from a reduction in their testosterone levels. However, recent heavy coverage of this topic in the national press has caused much concern and confusion about testosterone deficiency and it seems appropriate to discuss it.

Male menopause and testosterone deficiency are separate and distinct conditions. In physically normal men, the viropause/andropause syndrome occurs between forty and sixty and is a psychological disturbance. Testosterone deficiency occurs in men over sixty and is a physical (body chemical) abnormality.

Testosterone is one of the class of anabolic steroids that weight lifters and athletes use, although such people almost always use a steroid other than testosterone. Testosterone was first isolated from male urine in the 1930s. It was soon recognized as a mind-altering drug in that it produced aggressiveness in the recipients of the hormone. Hitler assigned some of his scientists the task of developing and using it to enhance the fighting nature of his army.

The male testes develop into maturity during adolescence. The gonads (sex glands or testes) begin their production of testosterone and spermatozoa at an average age of thirteen. At the time of maturity of the testes, the glands start secreting the hormone testosterone into the blood stream. The effects of this hormone are referred to as secondary sex changes and include characteristic male body hair, enlargement of the external genitalia, vocal cord changes (voice changes), appearance of a beard, male pattern muscle enlargement, and redistribution of body fat stores.

Under the influence of testosterone there are also mental changes. Childlike interests become more mature. A boy may become more introspective as he seeks to establish his identity. Most noticeable is the development of heterosexual interests and body functions. Boys become fascinated with females, especially their bodies, and begin masturbating; nocturnal emissions ("wet dreams") also start at this time.

The production of testosterone remains at a constant high level from adolescence until age fifty-five unless there is an illness or injury that affects the testes. These events are infrequent and seldom occur without the man being aware of them.

"I'm moody and miserable. I think I'm going through a mid-life crisis," said Earl Hunter, a forty-two-year-old who wanted help in relieving his increasing impotence. On examination I found he had small, soft testes. I ordered a blood test for testosterone deficiency.

At our next visit Earl brought his wide, Barbara, with him. I explained to both that Earl's testosterone level was below what was considered normal. I ordered further tests to establish a diagnosis of gonad failure–testosterone deficiency. When the tests came back positive, I talked to earl and his wife about testosterone replacement therapy, including its possible side effects. Together we decided to begin a program of regular testosterone injections for earl.

Testosterone deficiency before the age of fifty-five is very rare in normal healthy males. Earl's problem was due to bilateral (right and left) mumps of the testes at the age of thirteen. By mid-life his declining testosterone level had dropped precipitously. Regular injections of testosterone restored his libido.

Abnormal Deficiencies in Men under Fifty-Five

Men under the age of fifty-five who are healthy and have normal testes *do not have testosterone deficiency*. Only on rare occasions does an illness or accident produce a deficiency in these men.

The mumps virus, when contracted in adolescence, can occasionally affect one or both testes. This can occur only after the testes have already undergone some degree of maturity and, when it happens, often leaves the testes with some reduced activity for the remainder of the man's life. Few other infections or diseases impair testicular function. For example, a common infection localized to the scrotum, called epididymitis, does not interfere with the secretory function of the testes. Fortunately, cancer of the testes is rare and usually involves only one testis. Part of the treatment is removal of the affected testis, but the remaining testis usually continues to function normally.

Only one functioning testis is needed to produce adequate testosterone and sperm for reproduction. The reduced output of a single testis does not interfere with a man's sexuality.

In fetal life, the testes are in the abdomen and normally descend into the scrotum before birth. If this process is delayed, the testes remain in the abdomen and are referred to as "undescended testes." The undescended testes can be surgically treated and brought down into the scrotum. Depending on the patient's age (and other technical factors) at the time of surgery, the testis may or may not be functional.

Hernia operations do not affect testicular function unless there is an accidental disruption of the blood supply to the testes. The vasectomy only blocks the passage of sperm from the testis. It does not decrease the output of testosterone, so the amount secreted into the bloodstream is not reduced.

Severe accidental trauma to the scrotum (a wound or crushing) involving one or both testes will, of course, impair the gonadal function and can reduce or eliminate testosterone output.

Normal Deficiencies in Men over Fifty-Five

In contrast to the female ovaries, which, regardless of a woman's health, become totally inactive after menopause, the male gonads never become totally inactive. The blood levels of testosterone in healthy men start to decrease very gradually at about age fifty-five. There is some variation in the age at which this occurs as well as in the rate of decrease. The decrease is barely perceptible, even in blood tests, and is of no significance before age sixty.

In the normal, healthy man the descent of his blood testosterone level is very gradual. Low testosterone blood levels are seldom a cause of reduced sexuality in men under sixty-five. However, in more advanced ages, this normal gradual fall of testosterone may be enough to impair sexuality, although most healthy men are able to remain sexually active throughout their lives.

Abnormal Deficiencies in Men over Fifty-Five

Men over fifty-five are more likely to develop one of a number of diseases specific to the hormonal system or the genitalia that can abnormally lower their testosterone levels. Also, in some older men, especially those in poor health, the gradual normal fall-off of testosterone levels may, at some point, be enough to interfere with their sexuality.

Inadequate testosterone circulating in the blood can cause both mental and physical symptoms. The mental effects include a decrease in libido, a reduced feeling of well-being, and low energy level. Possible physical effects are muscle wasting, weakness, slow recovery from surgeries and illness, delicate bones (osteoporosis), and impairment of erectile function (impotence). The reduced sexuality experienced with low testosterone is then a combination of both the mental and physical effects.

Diagnosing Testosterone Deficiency

The patient's history is very important when diagnosing testosterone deficiency. Often the symptom that brings the patient to his doctor is a gradual development of sexual inadequacies, mostly erection difficulties. Less often it's reduced libido or orgasm delay. Additional symptoms may be similar to those found in depression: insomnia, dysphoria, apathy, withdrawal, fatigue, and psychosomatic symptoms.

When physicians suspect testosterone deficiency, they will ask about past illnesses and injuries that can reduce testosterone output in men under fifty-five (as described earlier in this chapter). They will also ask general health questions and inquire about any changes in sexuality.

There is a general physical examination with close

attention to the genitalia. The size of the testes, their softness or hardness, position in the scrotum, and tenderness are noted, as well as the presence of any abnormal masses. By way of a digital examination through the rectum, the prostate is evaluated. The prostate exam is important to rule out the possibility of carcinoma because, if there is prostate cancer, testosterone therapy must be withheld.

Laboratory testing of the urine and blood is needed to see if the symptoms are caused by some condition other than testosterone deficiency. The urinalysis can reveal a urinary infection and blood tests can show conditions such as anemia, thyroid malfunction, kidney and liver disease, and hyperlipidemia. A high lipid count (or high cholesterol) is a frequent cause of sexual inadequacy. A special study of the amount of testosterone in the blood is also usually performed. The prolactin level in the blood is also checked because, in a rare condition, this substance from the pituitary gland suppresses testicular output. It's especially important to rule out diabetes, because it is a common cause of impotence. Diabetes can be responsible for diseases of the arteries that supply the blood that hardens the penis.

If the result of the history, physical exam, and lab tests are positive for testosterone deficiency, then the physician will most likely prescribe a treatment of testosterone replacement.

Treatment of Testosterone Deficiency

Basically the treatment for testosterone deficiency is similar to the treatment for female estrogen deficiency: replacement. However, before replacement therapy is started there are other details that need attention. Underlying, contributing causes for the deficiency must be ruled out or treated. For example, diabetes must be treated with dietary management or medications such as insulin. The use of tobacco must be stopped.

Nicotine has a destructive effect on arteries and reduces blood flow to the penis. General health habits such as nutrition and exercise should be addressed.

Testosterone can be administered in one of several ways. Swallowing tablets is impractical because digestion destroys about half of the medication. Testosterone needs to be absorbed directly into the blood stream, bypassing the digestive system. Dissolvable tablets can be held in the mouth and absorbed into the blood stream via the mucous membranes under the tongue. At the present time, the best and most practical route is by injection of testosterone into the muscles. This is effective but inconvenient. The patient must go to a medical facility and receive a painful injection at two- to four-week intervals. Several research centers are conducting trials in the use of skin patches similar to the skin patches that deliver estrogen to menopausal women and nicotine to smokers who are trying to quit. It appears that testosterone administered by skin patches (placed around the scrotum) will soon be available.

During testosterone treatment the patient must be monitored regularly by his physician. Monitoring provides information useful in adjusting the dose to maximize the benefits and to minimize unpleasant side effects. The importance of this monitoring must be emphasized, because doses that are too large or administered for long periods of time can have serious and permanent side effects. The treatment goal is to find the smallest dose that will produce the desired response.

If reduced sexuality is caused by a testosterone

deficiency, testosterone replacement therapy will increase libido. The feeling of a need for sexual gratification is heightened and felt more frequently. (Testosterone has the same effect on women and is occasionally prescribed for this purpose.) Replacement therapy usually improves erections and orgasmic power as well. If these responses do not occur, there may be additional factors causing the problems or the diagnosis was incorrect.

Testosterone replacement produces psychological effects in addition to increasing the libido. The feeling of well-being returns, and some patients experience a feeling of euphoria. Because there is a frequent overlay of psychological elements when sexual inadequacy occurs, counseling is occasionally needed concomitant with the testosterone administration.

Testosterone can also have an addicting effect. The addictive features of testosterone (and other steroids) include enlargement of the muscles, feelings of euphoria and aggressiveness, and an increased sense of masculinity. To achieve these effects, large doses are required, creating a danger of an overdose and producing extremely negative side effects. For this reason the dispensing of testosterone must be closely regulated. (The harmful effects of the related androgens used for body building is widely recognized. The distribution of these drugs is poorly controlled.)

When testosterone or other steroids are used, the pituitary gland recognizes their presence and stops stimulating the testes to produce testosterone. This results in testicular atrophy as the testes decrease in size precipitously (in the gyms, it is referred to as "raisin nuts"). If the steroids are stopped, the testes do not return to their previous size or level of testosterone production. For this reason, testosterone therapy is being studied as a possible male contraceptive.

In large doses, testosterone and the other anabolic steroids also produce psychological side effects. In addition to aggression they produce irritability, which can be problematic in marital and other relationships. The irritability can also develop into bizarre behavior, called by users "'roid rages." This has some benefit for professional athletes such as football players because they increase their competitiveness and are stronger, more aggressive, and meaner.

Other physical side effects include benign liver tumors, transient hypertension, elevated serum cholesterol, lowered HDL (good cholesterol), acne, balding, jaundice, strokes, enlarged prostate, and occasional sudden death. These last are not common effects, but they are frequent and serious enough to be considered before prescribing testosterone or other anabolic steroids in large doses.

There can be confusion about proper treatment when male menopause and testosterone deficiency are diagnosed in the same man. Premature testosterone deficiency reduces a man's emotional well-being, which may precipitate or potentiate the viropause/andropause syndrome. Both conditions need to be treated. But there are additional problems when testosterone is prescribed as a treatment for male menopause. The psychological side effect of euphoria overrides the dysphoria of male menopause and masks the condition without curing it. The symptomatic treatment of the viropause/andropause syndrome with testosterone would be similar to treating it with alcohol. Both dispel unhappiness and substitute a temporary and artificial feeling of happiness. If the alcohol is withdrawn the man develops a hangover and is again unhappy, leading to the use of more alcohol. If artificially administered testosterone is withheld from the man experiencing male menopause, he will lose his feeling of well-being and masculinity. Physically, his muscles may get smaller and weaker. Overuse of testosterone causes atrophy (shrinking) of the testes, so the andropausal man will actually produce less testosterone. If a man experiencing the viropause/andropause syndrome is treated with testosterone when there is no actual testosterone deficiency, a true deficiency will develop, exhibiting all the symptoms described earlier.

CHAPTER 11

Myths and Truths about the Prostate

Radio and television commercials asking men whether they are experiencing such symptoms as difficulty in urination, getting up often to urinate at night, diminished urine streams, and pain during urination have become common. Meanwhile, heavy media coverage of celebrities such as Bill Bixby, who at age fifty-seven is in the final stages of prostate cancer, have made many men at mid-life apprehensive about their own possible prostate problems.

Men in their menopausal years hear tales about sexual dysfunction after prostate surgery from their fathers, older friends, and from the media and often become anxious about whether their own prostates are healthy. Most men do not have a clear concept of the role played by their secondary sex organs, and since they read and hear more about the prostate than the other two organs (the seminal vesicles and the epididymis), they often become fearful about whether they have or soon will have prostate difficulties. Because these fears are so widespread and are often based on misinformation, it is beneficial to know the truth about the prostate.

The prostate gland is a solid (not hollow) structure surrounding the urethra located at the base of the urinary bladder in men. The healthy adult prostate is the size and shape of an English walnut. The role played by the prostate in sexual intercourse is relatively minor. Its only function is to supply and secrete into the urethra, a lubricant for intercourse. This lubricating fluid also acts as a vehicle for sperm during ejaculation.

The three most common disorders of the prostate are infections, enlargement (benign prostatic hypertrophy), and cancer. Infections occur commonly at all adult ages. Mild infections cause mild to moderate discomfort in the pelvis and anal area. With more severe infections, there is pain in the same areas associated with fever. The infection responds well but slowly to antibiotics. It's not unusual for prostate infections to require several months of treatment. Mild infections occur quite often and can become chronic. Fortunately, infections are not usually transmitted to sexual partners and do not impair sexual function. In rare cases, bacteria from the prostate can enter the bloodstream, causing a serious illness requiring hospitalization and intense care. Infections impair sexuality only if severe or if the patient allows them to become a source of psychological significance.

The prostate of every man undergoes gradual progressive enlargement as he grows older. Enlargement begins in mid-life but rarely causes problems or symptoms until later in life. The age of onset of prostate enlargement and the rate of progression are both variable. Usually prostate enlargement produces no symptoms for several years. Eventually there are one or more symptoms of urinary obstruction: more frequent day time urination, getting up at night to empty the bladder, hesitancy in starting urination, small-caliber stream, less force of the stream, and dribbling after voiding. No treatment is necessary unless these symptoms become too much of a nuisance, there is complete obstruction, or the condition leads to urinary infection.

Benign prostate enlargement can be treated either medically or surgically. The medical treatment includes oral medication to shrink the size of the prostate gland. It requires six months to a year to determine its effectiveness. Medication can control enlargement, but it is not a cure.

Surgical correction of enlarged prostates has been used for decades. The surgery is performed in the hospital with either general or a spinal anesthesia. The urologist passes an optical instrument through the urethra and visualizes the obstructing prostate tissue. The doctor then removes the obstructing tissues. Patients often refer to the procedure as a "ream job" or "roto-rooter." The operation is almost always successful but does have one side effect: retrograde ejaculation.

This occurs because during prostate surgery the nerve and muscle structures are disturbed and, as a consequence, ejaculation is altered. Thus during climax the semen flow direction is reversed. The semen flows into the bladder instead of squirting from the urethra. It is comforting to know that this does not diminish the wonderful sensation of orgasm for the man, and because the upper two-thirds of a woman's vagina has no sensory nerves, the man's partner experiences no change in her sensations either with retrograde ejaculation. Some couples even consider this a change for the better—less "mopping up" is needed after ejaculation.

A man may require removal of the obstructing prostate tissue if he has a benign disease of the prostate. This can be occasionally required to relieve obstruction during a man's fifties. Happily the procedure does not cause impotence.

Some men are concerned about the relationship between vasectomies for sterilization and various diseases including prostate disorders and about the effect of vasectomies on sexuality. For many years reports by the media have suggested vasectomy increases the risk of this or that disease. However, most good scientific research agrees vasectomies do not cause abnormalities in other parts of the body. A vasectomy obstructs the passage of sperm. It doesn't alter the production of testosterone nor does it interfere with the flow of testosterone into the bloodstream. Consequently, surgical vasectomies do not impair sexuality either directly or indirectly.

A man already fearful about his mid-life sexuality and experiencing the viropause/andropause syndrome may become obsessed with the idea that he has diseases of the prostate. He will vigilantly watch himself for signs of obstruction. One or two visits to the doctor can be very reassuring and eliminate this element of the viropause/andropause syndrome.

Prostate cancer is common. Twenty-three percent of cancers that start in men start in the prostate. Fortunately, only twelve percent of cancer deaths are of the prostate. (The incidence of lung cancer is eighteen percent, but it is responsible for thirty-four percent of the deaths.) Deaths from cancer of the prostate and colon are almost equal in number in the United States (28,982 and 28,111, respectively). As with most cancer, early detection is the most important determinant in the outcome—cure or death.

When Robert levy, age fifty-seven, came to my office for his annual examination, I found a significantly elevated PSA level. Though the problem is far more common in men beyond the andropausal age, my follow-up diagnostic evaluation unfortunately established that Robert had prostate cancer.

Robert told me his greatest fear was impotence. After reassuring him that we now have improved techniques for this procedure, techniques that better the chances of sparing the nerves that are needed to produce an erection, I recommended tat he make an immediate appointment with a urologist.

He and the urologist decided that he best approach to curing the disease was the surgical removal of the prostate. Fortunately, Robert's operation was successful not only in removing the cancer, but also in not damaging the nerves needed for penile erection.

For those patients who are left impotent after surgery, counseling is available to select a method of artificially creating satisfactory erections.

There is increasing interest in the subject of prostate carcinoma, both by physicians and their patients, and there appears to be an increasing incidence of this cancer. Researchers are not in agreement as to why this is. Some of them believe it is a real increase, others that it is not. Perhaps because of better means of making early diagnosis, men are living longer and other serious diseases are successfully recognized and treated, and so on.

The media has popularized a blood test used for detecting prostate cancer, the PSA. All men have Prostatic

Specific Antigen in their blood. The level increases in the presence of prostate disease. It also goes up in the presence of prostate enlargement (hypertrophy), and it goes up even more when there is cancer in the organ. Unfortunately, this difference is not always great enough to distinguish between the two conditions.

The PSA test does not have a good record for sensitivity or specificity. Good sensitivity means a test has few false negatives. Good specificity means it has few false positives. The evaluation of these two characteristics of the test shows a false positive rate of thirty-seven to forty percent and a false negative rate of forty to forty-five percent when there is no other evidence of prostate cancer. This is a pretty poor showing. In order for a test to be useful to the physician and patient, it should produce a false result less than ten percent of the time.

When the test is falsely negative for cancer, the patient may become too complacent. He may delay or omit having regular examinations for the disease; he may even ignore symptoms that suggest possible cancer growth. When a test result is negative, the physician may minimize other suggestive evidence of carcinoma.

When the test is falsely positive, of course, the patient becomes alarmed and worries. The physician is obliged to set in motion a series of diagnostic procedures, referral to a urologist, ultrasound studies, biopsies, and possibly more unnecessary expenditures of time and money.

For these and other more complex reasons the PSA hasn't been completely embraced by the medical community. The big question remains: Should it be used as a screening test—should every male over a certain age have the test at regular intervals in the absence of any other symptoms or physical findings of prostate carcinoma?

Despite the problems with the results of this test, it is very easy for the physician to add PSA to the list of blood tests along with cholesterol, blood sugar, and others. I suspect that it will become a routine test, but patients should be aware of he limitations of the PSA. Men should also be aware that prostate cancer rarely shows early warning symptoms such as difficulty in urination. The rectal exam remains the mainstay in early detection. It has survived the test of time and can often detect cancer of the rectum as well.

Breast and prostate cancers have some characteristics in common: neither produce any early symptoms; both must be detected early to improve cure rates; there is no one way to ensure early detection. For these very reasons every means available must be used to improve survival rates. Women do self-examinations monthly, have mammography and physicians' examinations annually. Men likewise should have rectal prostate examinations yearly and the PSA blood test regularly.

Prostate cancer occasionally begins in mid-life but almost always produces no symptoms until later life and generally is not fatal until old age. It grows slowly, and only in advanced cases does it spread to other parts of the body.

One of the most feared surgical procedures for prostate cancer is castration. Most men consider castration the ultimate insult to the body and to masculinity. However, even though castration does produce sterility, it does not always reduce sexuality or cause impotence.

Cure rates with surgery and/or chemotherapy are high. For advanced malignancy of the prostate we use surgery, chemotherapy, and radiation. These therapies alter sexual function for many men. Fortunately, even with extensive procedures we now have ways to artificially restore potency, allowing for gratifying sexual functioning.

Men in their andropausal years, concerned about prostate problems, can become overly apprehensive about the effects of cancer surgery on sexuality and often fear the possibility of their own impotency. This fear may precipitate the male menopause syndrome or intensify it. It can also become a barrier to recovery from the condition. In a man who has an underlying mental disorder such as anxiety or depression, prostate surgery can trigger erectile failures. These underlying psychological conditions must be treated to correct the problem of impotency. Most of the sexual problems can be prevented by explanations and counseling by the urologist before surgery. For some patients who are extremely anxious, additional visits may be required after the surgery.

CHAPTER 12

When Professional Help Is Needed

A new patient of mine, Allen Samuelson, age fifty-nine, lived in a city forty-five miles away. When he made the appointment the receptionist asked if he wanted a general history and physical examination. He declined, saying, "I just want an office visit to see about getting a prescription."

Allen had a professional degree and was an elected official in the city where he lived. He told me he didn't want to see his own doctor for his problem because, "It's a small town and everybody knows everything about everybody." He then asked me for a prescription for an antidepressant. He was certain he had a depression disorder.

Two weeks previously, Allen had called his brother for advice. He had been feeling "depressed" for several months and it was gradually getting worse. He knew his brother had been diagnosed as having a depression disorder and the prescribed medication had made him "his old self again." Allen was aware that depression runs in families. The brother had responded to Allen by saying, "It sure sounds like depression. You had better see a doctor and get a prescription."

Allen was emphatic that he didn't want to see a psychiatrist or psychologist in his hometown. He was certain of his own diagnosis and treatment. He was obviously annoyed when I told him he would have to come in again for a longer visit to establish a diagnosis and to select an appropriate treatment. But he reluctantly agreed to the suggestion and signed a release for his hometown physician to send the record of his last examination and laboratory results.

I was assured by his medical record there were no physical abnormalities that could mimic depression and decided to search further. When he returned, he told me about his deepening distress. He had tried to dispel his unhappiness by adjusting his work schedule and changing his lifestyle, but his efforts had not been successful. It became apparent by the end of the hour that Allen did not have a depression disorder. There had been no changes in his eating or sleeping habits, no drop in his energy level, no thoughts of suicide, no problems with concentration, and no change in libido.

The other history he related to me suggested he was experiencing male menopause. I discussed this probable diagnosis and gave him material to read at home about depression and andropause. When he returned for his third and final appointment he agreed with the diagnosis and wanted advice for getting counseling. I gave him the names and phone numbers of three therapists in my area. I asked him to call me after he had made his selection so I could arrange the referral. A few days later he called and I arranged an appointment.

Six weeks later I received a referral report from the psychiatrist. He agreed with my diagnosis and told me Allen was making good progress.

When a man in his middle years becomes unhappy for no obvious or apparent external reason, when the cause is not physical, when feelings of discontent predominate, and when he is unable to shake these feelings by his own efforts, it is a sign that something serious is wrong. When the andropausal male's own efforts to relieve the distress he feels are unsuccessful, he obviously needs help. He may seek it first from friends and family. If their help is inadequate, he will, if he is wise, seek professional counsel. Early diagnosis helps shorten the time required to restore an andropausal man's health. It is hoped that any man who has uncontrollable symptoms of male menopause will realize that something is wrong early and will seek help right away. The briefer the illness, the less damage the man or his family will suffer. In this time of stress and personal agony, he may say and do hurtful things that can damage others and leave him with strong feelings of guilt even after his recovery. Getting such help is especially urgent if the man's condition is causing his personal relationships to erode—if he is having serious problems with his family at home or his colleagues at work. It is also urgent if there is any disability associated with the syndrome. The disability may be apparent as an impairment of his work performance. It may also manifest itself in drinking problems, insomnia, or lack of energy.

Because male menopause can be of long duration and can, unfortunately, become chronic or irreversible, getting professional help makes good sense. Life is too short to waste months or years in a state of discontent. Ironically, the realization that one's time is limited and that life is shorter than one had imagined can be emotionally paralyzing.

Fortunately, many men feel comfortable talking to their physician, and most primary physicians are acquainted with the work of local counselors and can recommend one or more. Of course, the telephone yellow pages can provide a list of counselors, but choosing one from such a list can present problems. In large cities there may be too many listed and in small communities too few listed to make an easy choice. In addition, the listings may not be specific enough to provide sufficient guidance.

Selecting a Counselor

Most primary physicians, general practitioners, family physicians, and internists are trained and skilled in psychology, so referral to a therapist often is not needed. With the changes in health care patterns, more and more patients will develop a doctor–patient relationship with one of these primary physicians. A physician can be a viable choice for counseling if the symptoms are not too severe and if the doctor is agreeable. Many times when I have suggested to patients they would benefit from a referral to a counselor their response has been, "Can't you do it? I'd rather see you than someone new." I have usually agreed and the outcome has been satisfactory.

However, if a mental health professional is needed or desired, there are many from which to choose. Counselors may be listed as marriage, family, or individual therapists; they may be Christian counselors, transactional counselors, group counselors, psychiatrists, or psychologists. They may be listed according to their degree: B.A., B.S., M.A., M.D.,

WHEN PROFESSIONAL HELP IS NEEDED

M.S., or Ph.D. Other initials that follow their names might include L.C.P., L.C.S.W.V., L.M.C.C., L.M.F.T., or L.P.C., indicating their training and/or licenses. The person who attempts to select a counselor may find this a bewildering thicket of labels. If so, the primary physician may be able to provide names of well-qualified counselors.

Tom Fuller, a fifty-seven-year-old skilled workman came to my office concerned that he might have prostate cancer. His uncle was in the terminal stage of prostate cancer and Tom's worry about it was intensified by his own need to get up twice nightly to empty his bladder. His exam and lab test did not suggest cancer; however, his history and lab tests were abnormal.

The family history included the death of another uncle due to complications of alcoholism. As part of the routine dietary history, I said, "Tell me about your alcohol intake—how much, how often, and what?" His answer was, "Oh, not too much. After work I stop with two of the guys who work for me and have a few beers [on direct questioning, it was four or five], and when I get home my wife and I have a couple of mixed drinks. Sometimes [five or six nights per week] after the evening meal I watch TV and have some wine [three glasses]." He assured me, "I never drink at work or by myself."

I suggested this was an excessive alcohol intake and asked how long he had been drinking this much. It was then the really significant history surfaced. About twenty months earlier he had had a financial problem. His shop had been busy and taking in good profits, but he hadn't saved enough to pay his taxes. He had to borrow a rather large amount from the bank. When he completed the loan application forms, he realized his entire financial condition was in bad shape. He started mulling about his future, his ability to set aside funds for retirement, and paying off the mortgages on his home and his shop.

It was about the same time that Tom developed the very annoying habit of waking around 2:00 A.M. and not being able to return to sleep (a common sleep pattern in those who drink excessively). This had been going on for those twenty months. While he was awake and tossing around in bed, he worried about his financial status, which soon led to his worrying about other aspects of his life. His daytime energy level decreased, which he attributed to his lack of sleep. He grew dissatisfied with his limited achievements and with himself in general. He became irritable. One of his good employees quit after a series of arguments. His daughter's family stopped visiting regularly. His wife pointed out to him, "It's no wonder, the way you always dig them about everything." He responded to her comments with intense anger followed by a sense of guilt.

Tom told himself the after-work beers with the employees were a good idea because they showed he was a congenial boss, but he also knew the beer relieved the "bad feeling" he was having every day while at work. He soon realized that continuing the alcohol in the evening "kept the bad feelings away." Eight months earlier he decided he was drinking too much and quit cold turkey. It didn't work. He became even more cranky and started feeling jittery. He returned to his previous drinking pattern after nine days of abstinence.

Since several of his blood tests were abnormal, we discussed the findings and I observed they looked as though he was drinking even more than he had reported. He admitted that maybe he was. I told him that his liver function tests indicated early damage. This impressed him, as his alcoholic uncle had liver disease.

After taking more history, I was able to rule out a depression disorder. I concluded he was indeed suffering the miseries of male menopause. We talked about this and I gave him material on the subject to take home and read. I strongly advised professional counseling. He needed it for treatment of both male menopause and alcoholism.

When he returned the following week, I offered to arrange admittance to a local facility specializing in the treatment of alcoholism, but he preferred to try quitting on his own with help from a counselor. He had talked to a relative and two friends who had had successful experiences with counselors and had already selected a therapist. I knew the therapist because I had referred other patients to him and they had been helped, some with male menopause, others with alcoholism, and some with both.

I am hopeful that next year Tom will report successful abstinence and a happier outlook for his future and will have re-established good relationships with his family. In addition he will probably be getting better sleep and not having to empty his bladder so often during the night. If he does abstain from alcohol, his liver tests could return to normal. Full liver recovery can be achieved if the alcohol damage is not too extensive.

Considering the particular symptoms of male menopause is a way to narrow the choices of a proper counselor. If marital problems are an important part of the complex, a marriage counselor would be a good choice to begin with. If there is impaired work performance, perhaps the employer or the firm he works for may have a counselor who could be consulted. Or it could be possible to contact a consultant whose expertise is stress management, communications, or employment assistance. If alcohol or other drugs are part of the problem, an experienced substance abuse counselor would be an appropriate choice. Consulting a psychiatrist is recommended if the individual is suffering from depression or if he has a past history of mental disturbance. A psychiatrist is also a good choice if psychosomatic symptoms such as headaches, indigestion, sexual dysfunction, or extreme fatigue are a part of the problem.

It is very important to find a counselor who acknowledges that the male menopause is a medical entity and who has experience in treating this disorder. If only the symptoms are treated—which might be the case if the counselor had limited familiarity with the viropausal/andropausal condition—the outcome can be unsatisfactory. The elimination of one symptom, for example, drug abuse, may simply provoke another, such as a psychosomatic illness, to surface. The process could be compared to treating appendicitis by removing the pain. Analgesics can stop the pain of an attack, but surgical removal of the appendix is necessary to effect a cure.

Talking to other individuals who themselves have had counseling can help in making a selection. Friends, relatives, and acquaintances are often willing to discuss their experiences with therapy. One needs to remember, however, that a particular therapist's approach to a psychological problem may suit one person but not another. And different conditions may require quite different methods of treatment.

A call to the local or county medical society is another way to learn about counselors. Medical societies will not recommend one therapist, but they will give the names of several in the area. Medical schools are also a good source of information about counselors. In addition to names, they can provide background information about the education and experience of counselors in a particular area. Professional medical organizations can provide objective information and lists of counselors one can choose from.

People who have a religious affiliation or who are familiar with a particular church might consider the counseling services available through the church. Part of the professional training in seminaries includes courses in counseling and psychology. Many rabbis, priests, and ministers are excellent counselors.

Choosing a therapist is a good deal like choosing a friend. The two personalities—patient's and therapist's—should be complementary. Positive feelings about each other should emerge early in the relationship. (It should be noted that anyone who has selected a counselor should be willing to give counseling a chance. To have doubts about the value of therapy is to severely limit the possibilities that it will be effective.) Trust and respect are essential. It is most important that the patient feels the counselor and the counselor's approach to be right and comfortable. Patients who have reservations after the first or second visit should consider selecting another counselor and not feel that to do so would be a waste of money. Neither the patient nor the counselor benefits from continuing when the first few sessions have been unproductive. Counselors are in the profession because they have a personal as well as a professional commitment to helping, and they need to know that they are successful with their clients. In a way, a counselor must become a friend. Just as the first person one meets in a new community may not turn out to be a close friend, so the first counselor one consults may not turn out to be the best therapist for that man.

What to Expect

As to what to expect during counseling, my comments are intentionally limited for the following reason: Individual therapists have their own distinct manner of working with their clients. What is successful for one may not work for another. To try to describe what can be expected in therapy would be to set standards or criteria that the patient might use in judging his therapist. No one can really determine the effectiveness of a counselor except the patient himself. A satisfactory outcome for any medical treatment depends a great deal on the patient's confidence in the doctor and the treatment. Having preconceived expectations about how a counselor might proceed can be a hindrance.

I can tell you that most treatment is primarily by means of guided discussion. The therapist asks questions to discover the patient's thoughts and ideas. The patient will find some of his ideas reinforced and others diminished. Therapists do not express any moral judgments and they make few judgmental observations. Their function is to allow the patient to explore ideas and options openly.

A counselor may ask his patient to consult a physician in order to rule out the possibility of physical problems, such as thyroid or other endocrine disorders, that might affect his psychological condition. It is also possible for the counselor to consider whether there is an underlying mental disorder, such as depression or chronic anxiety. Psychiatrists are also M.D.s, so a counselor who is also a psychiatrist will be able to diagnose and treat these conditions with medication; other counselors may refer their patients to a psychiatrist for diagnosis if a mental disorder needing medication is suspected.

The length of time that therapy requires to alleviate male menopausal symptoms varies greatly. It may be as brief as two weeks—two sessions perhaps—or as long as a year. Usually, though, results can be achieved in a few months. As with other illnesses, the severity of the condition dictates the duration and intensity of the treatment. If the patient is deeply disturbed or has complicating conditions, such as severe depression, the course of treatment will be longer. In contrast, if the patient is basically stable and there are no complicating factors, only a few counseling sessions may be needed. It is also important to know that support from family and friends can help shorten the period needed for therapy.

A counselor's particular mode of treatment determines somewhat how many visits will be appropriate. Usually the visits will be scheduled at weekly intervals and will last about an hour each. After the first few visits, the interval between sessions is sometimes extended from every week to every two to four weeks.

As discussed in Chapter 6, viropausal/andropausal men do not necessarily need to seek professional help, and most do not. However, when self-help does not relieve the problems and when his primary physician can't help, a counselor is a very valuable resource, and the man who doesn't find relief for his symptoms should not hesitate to consult one. It is well worth the cost and effort. Untreated, male menopause can have profound and long lasting effects on a man's life.

CHAPTER 13

Most Frequently Asked Questions about Male Menopause

What is the male menopause?
It is a biological and biochemical condition that has psychological, physical, and emotional components. Viropause/andropause is a naturally occurring psychological state that occurs in men's middle years, producing feelings of unhappiness and undermining men's sense of self-worth, identity, and competence.

At what age does the viropause/andropause syndrome occur?
The onset of male menopause is generally between the ages of forty and sixty; some men, probably less than five percent, start in their late thirties, and another ten percent start in their sixties.

Does a woman's menopause occur at the same age as a man's andropause?
Yes, approximately. Most women become menopausal between the ages of forty-five and fifty-five with eight percent starting earlier, some as early as thirty-eight.

How long does male menopause last?
If untreated, it can last anywhere from a few days to several years. A very small percentage of men never recover.

What are some of the physical symptoms of the male menopause syndrome?
They include health factors that can become increasingly important after fifty. These include diabetes, hypertension, heart disease, arteriosclerosis (resulting in decreased blood flow to the penis), some lessening of sexuality, and natural mid-life aging processes.

What are the causes of the male menopause syndrome?
Disappointment in goals not achieved, fears about aging, sexual inadequacy, financial insecurity, retirement, and stress.

Does retirement bring on male menopause?
The fears and misgivings concerning retirement may be a causal factor.

How is the andropause syndrome related to sexuality?
It's related in two ways: fears about decreasing sexuality can be a cause of andropause, and andropausal symptoms can affect sexuality.

Is sexual deficiency a cause of male menopause?
When a man becomes aware of sexual deficiencies, he feels inadequate and starts worrying about the possibility of future reduction in his sexuality, which leads to dysphoria.

Do all men experiencing male menopause have serious problems?
No. Fifteen percent have problems serious enough to be considered ill. Probably fewer than half have symptoms that can be considered disabling. The rest have "bad spells" of days or weeks.

How does a man know he is entering male menopause?
He becomes less happy and has pervasive feelings of anxiety, discontent, and worry.

How does the anxiety of male menopause feel?
Nervous, restless, apprehensive, and sometimes "shaky inside."

Can this dysphoria (unhappiness) be caused by other things?
Yes. Some physical illnesses, such as hormonal diseases and deficiencies, can mimic male menopause.

Is depression the same as the viropause/andropause syndrome?
No. The unhappiness of depression is like that of male menopause, but the depressed person experiences additional symptoms such as change of eating and sleeping patterns, hopelessness, a feeling of worthlessness, and reduced libido. A professional evaluation may be required to

distinguish between the two. Depression responds favorably to anti-depressive medication while andropause may not.

Couldn't a man have both the andropause syndrome and depression?
Yes. This would require professional assessment and treatment.

We all have bad days when we're unhappy. Why is the unhappiness associated with male menopause different?
In male menopause a man's "down" mood increases and persists.

How does physical aging affect male menopause?
The man experiencing male menopause perceives early signs of aging, such as hair loss or a developing paunch, as a predictor of disastrous and rapid body deterioration.

And does male menopause affect a man's sexuality?
After fifty, though physical problems such as diabetes, heart disease, high cholesterol, hypertension, or restricted blood flow to the penis, and because most sexuality is mentally motivated, the psychological symptoms of the viropause/andropause syndrome, which include unhappiness and anxiety, can impair sexual functions like libido, erections, and orgasm.

Don't men always have a high libido?
Yes, but the normal level does vary over a lifetime. Male libido reaches a peak in the late twenties and early thirties then very slowly but definitely wanes for the next two

decades of life. However, libido never totally disappears in the healthy male.

Are women's libido patterns similar to men's?
No. Women's libidos definitely increase in their menopausal years, at the same time andropausal men's libidos are decreasing. This creates an unfortunate disparity of libido for many couples.

How can male menopause affect one's libido?
Feelings of dysphoria or anxiety can crowd out, and sometimes eradicate, the normal loving and erotic thoughts that underlie the sex drive.

What can a couple do about the disparity in libido?
If there is good and healthy communication channel between the two they can make appropriate adjustments.

What's the most common form of sexual dysfunction associated with male menopause?
Erection failures: Total inability to get an erection, loss of erection during thrusting, or a partial erection that is adequate but less firm than previously. These are common occurrences and considered normal when they occur sporatically in the late forties and fifties. Erection problems are only considered abnormal at this stage in life if there is total loss of erectile power (impotence) every time. However, organic factors are much more significant in men over fifty-five than had previously been thought.

Why does sexual dysfunction cause the viropause/andropause syndrome?

Sexual dysfunction can cause abnormal fear, which is one
of the basic components in the establishment of andropause: fear that sexual dysfunction will get progressively
worse, fear that the dysfunction is a significant sign of generalized physical aging, and fear that a lowered libido will
cause the man's wife to seek a new lover.

**How does a man's sexual dysfunction disrupt the mari-
tal relationship?**
Because of his fear of failure, a man may avoid sexual activity with his wife. This is directly disruptive because of
the absence of a physical expression of the couple's love
and an indirect disruption if the wife believes incorrectly
that the sexual avoidance indicates the man is having an
affair.

**How do men react to the bad feelings and anxiety asso-
ciated with male menopause?**
There are many possible responses: losing interest in home,
family, and work; irritability, crankiness, shortened temper,
unreasonableness, impatience; and change in behavior.

**How does a man's behavior change in response to male
menopause?**
Behavioral changes include making inappropriate decisions
about expenditures, losing interest in hobbies, dropping old
friendships, finding new and younger friends, increasing
the use of alcohol and other drugs, wearing younger clothing and hair styles, finding an interest in younger women,
taking up inappropriate exercise or sports.

How does male menopause affect the man's personal

relationships?
It has a disruptive effect on relationships at home. Because he is unreasonable and cranky, communications break down. He may become verbally combative and say things he will later regret.

Are extramarital affairs frequent during the viropausal/andropausal years?
Yes. For various reasons the man in andropause is often susceptible. He may erroneously suspect his unhappiness is boredom or a dissatisfaction with his wife, so he seeks a new outlet for female companionship and sex.

How does male menopause affect sexual performance?
Andropause tends to decrease sexual performance. However, a new female partner can mentally and physically stimulate the andropausal man so that his sexual prowess is temporarily raised to the level he experienced in his youth. As the newness wears off there is usually a return to the previous inadequacies. This is very disappointing and can deepen the andropause.

Does male menopause increase the separation, divorce, and remarriage rate?
It probably does, although there are no current research figures to support this.

How does the viropause/andropause syndrome affect the man's work relationships?
Because of his unpleasantness he loses friends or his friends avoid him. He may become less productive because of an impairment in his relationships.

How does male menopause decrease work productivity?
Insomnia, excessive alcohol consumption, and preoccupation with troubles reduce mental acuity and cause physical fatigue that detract from productive work.

Does testosterone deficiency cause male menopause?
Not in a healthy man. There is very rarely a precipitous testosterone decrease in physically healthy men under age fifty-five. In men fifty-five to sixty there is a minimal decrease, mostly of free testosterone, but not enough to impair sexual function or cause psychological effects. The percentage of men with lowered testosterone goes up with advancing age over sixty-five.

What causes testosterone deficiency in men under sixty?
A very small percentage of men under sixty have a physical abnormality of the pituitary gland or testes that can cause a testosterone deficiency. For these men, there is usually a history of testicular illness (mumps, injury, or accidental castration) or both testes are absent or very small.

How is a testosterone deficiency diagnosed?
Urine tests have been used in the past, but now a blood test is used along with a patient history and physical examination.

Should all men over sixty-five be tested for testosterone deficiency?
Only if they are having symptoms of reduced sexuality, a decrease in their feeling of well-being, and their physician suspects a deficiency.

What is the treatment for testosterone deficiency?
In the rare cases that occur, the treatment is administration of testosterone by injection at two- to four-week intervals or by testosterone tablets placed under the tongue. Testosterone patches may become available in the future.

Are there side effects from testosterone treatments?
Yes, but usually not severe or irreversible if given in the appropriate doses for a limited time by an ethical physician. The psychological effects of overdose include excessive aggression and belligerence and, in extreme cases, uncontrollable rages. The physical side effects of an overdose are enlarged muscles, oily skin, increased appetite, excessive libido, and hair follicle depletion of the scalp. Medical side effects include hypertension, liver diseases, decreased size and activity of the testes, and sterility.

How can a man help himself when he realizes he's experiencing male menopause?
By seeing a doctor about physical complaints and by re-evaluating and reordering his life. This means setting realistic goals, establishing appropriate priorities, and examining his values.

What percentage of andropausal men require treatment?
Only the most severely disturbed need professional guidance—probably about fifteen percent of all men. An additional fifteen percent will recognize their andropausal condition and treat it themselves or recover with help from family or friends. There are no accurate figures available. The subject needs more research.

CHAPTER 13

When should the man experiencing male menopause seek professional help?

When there are physical symptoms, when it's destroying his personal relationships, when the symptoms are growing progressively worse, when he begins developing a dependence on alcohol or other chemicals, or when it seems to him that his own efforts are inadequate.

What does the future hold for a man experiencing male menopause?

When he has recovered he will become happier and be more contented than ever before in his life. He will adapt to adversity better and no longer be fearful of the future.

Glossary

ACUITY: Clarity or clearness.

ADRENAL: A gland situated near the kidney.

AGORAPHOBIA: Intense, irrational fear of open spaces. A complex phobic disorder characterized by marked fear of being alone or of public places where escape would be difficult or help might be unavailable.

ANABOLIC: Constructive metabolic process by which organisms convert substances into other components.

ANALGESIC: Any medication that reduces or eliminates pain.

ANDROIDAL HORMONES: Chemicals producing manlike characteristics.

ANDROPAUSE: Male menopause; a medically defined dysphoria or unease that occurs in men usually between the ages of forty and sixty.

ANTICHOLENERGICS: Chemicals that block certain nerves.

ANTIHISTAMINE: A drug used to reduce histamine production in allergies and colds.

ANXIETY: Apprehension, tension, or uneasiness from anticipation of danger, the source of which is largely unknown or unrecognized.

ATROPHY: A wasting away; a diminution in the size of a cell, tissue or organ.

BIOLOGICAL: Pertaining to the phenomenon of life and living

organisms in general.

CASTRATION: Removal of the gonads (male - testes, female - ovaries).

CEREBRAL: Pertaining to the main portion of the brain.

CHRONIC: Persisting over a long period of time.

CIRRHOSIS: Liver disease characterized pathologically by loss of the normal lobular architecture, with fibrosis and nodular regeneration.

CLIMACTERIC: A period in life at the termination of the reproductive cycle when endocrine, somatic and psychic changes occur.

CLIMAX: The acme, or period of greatest intensity in sexual excitement; orgasm.

CLINICAL: Pertaining to actual observation and treatment of patients, as distinguished from theoretical or basic sciences.

CLITORIS: A small, elongated, erectile body, situated at the upper end of the vulva of the female external genitalia, corresponding to the male penis.

COITUS: Sexual intercourse achieved by insertion of a man's penis into a woman's vagina.

COLLAGEN: The protein substance of the white fibers of skin, tendon, bone and cartilage.

COPULATION: Sexual intercourse.

CORPUS LUTEUM: A reddish yellow mass (tissue) that forms from the rupture of the follicle of a woman's ovary.

COUNSELOR: One who discusses, deliberates, and gives advice.

DEPRESSION: A psychiatric syndrome consisting of dejected mood, psychomotor retardation, insomnia, weight change, sometimes with guilt feelings and somatic preoccupation, often of exaggerated proportions.

DIAGNOSTIC: Distinctive of a disease; a symptom serving as supporting evidence in a diagnosis.

DIHYDROTESTOSTERONE: A powerful androgenic (masculine characteristics) hormone formed in peripheral tissue (tissue other than the testes) by the action on testosterone; is responsible for development of most secondary characteristics at puberty and for adult male sexual functions.

DILATORY: Pertaining to dilation; causing to make wider or to expand.

DYSFUNCTIONAL: Impaired functioning of a body system or organ.

DYSPAREUNIA: Difficult or painful sexual intercourse.

DYSPHORIA: Disquiet, restlessness, malaise, unpleasant mood.

EGO: A psychoanalytic theory concerning the psychological segment of the personality. The self; the individual as aware of himself (colloq). EGOTISM, conceit.

EJACULATE: To suddenly expel semen in the male orgasm.

EJACULATION: The sudden expulsion of semen in male orgasm.

ELECTROCARDIOGRAM: A graphic tracing of the variations in electrical activity of the heart muscle.

ENDOCRINE: Secreting internally; applied to organs whose function is to secrete into the blood a substance (hormone) that has a specific effect on another organ.

EQUANIMITY: Quality of remaining calm and undisturbed, evenness of mind or temper; composure.

ERECTILE: Capable of erection.

ERECTION: The condition of being made rigid and elevated, as the penis when filled with blood.

EROTIC: Charged with sexual feeling; pertaining to sexual desire.

ESTROGEN: A female hormone formed in the ovary.

ETIOLOGY: The study of factors that cause disease; the cause(s) or origin of a disease or disorder.

EUPHORIA: An exaggerated feeling of physical and mental well being, especially when not justified by external reality.

FERTILE: Capable of reproducing.

FOREPLAY: The sexually stimulating, usually pleasurable activity preceding sexual intercourse.

GASTROINTESTINAL: Pertaining to or communicating with the stomach and the intestine.

GENITALIA: The various internal and external organs concerned with reproduction.

GERIATRIC: Pertaining to the aged and their characteristic afflictions.

GONAD: An organ that produces mature sperm (the male testis) or egg (the female ovary).

GYN: Abbreviation for gynecologic; pertaining to or affecting the female reproductive tract.

GYNECOLOGICAL: Pertaining to or affecting the female reproductive tract.

HDL: High density lipoprotein. The "good cholesterol."

HORMONE: A chemical substance, produced in the body by an organ or cells of an organ which has specific regulatory effect on the activity of a certain organ; endocrine.

HOT FLASHES: A sudden brief flushing and sensation of heat caused by dilation of skin capillaries, usually associated with menopausal endocrine imbalance.

HYPERPROLACTINEMIA: Increased levels of prolactin, a hormone secreted by the pituitary into the blood.

HYPERTENSION: Persistently high pressure in the arteries.

HYSTERECTOMY: Surgical removal of the uterus.

IMPOTENCE: Lack of power, chiefly of copulative power in the male; incapable of sexual intercourse.

INSOMNIA: Inability to sleep; unable to sleep.

INTERCOURSE: Coitus; sexual joining of male and female.

INTROMISSION: The insertion of the penis into the vagina in copulation.

L.C.P.: Licensed clinical psychologist.

L.C.S.W.: Licensed clinical social worker.

L.M.F.T.: Licensed marriage family counselor.

L.P.C.: Licensed professional counselor.

LASSITUDE: A state of exhaustion or torpor.

LETHARGIC: Pertaining to abnormal drowsiness or stupor.

LIBIDO: Sexual desire; manifestation of the sexual drive.

LIPID: Fats and fat-like substances.

M.F.C.C.: Marriage family child counselor.

M.S.: Master of science degree.

MALAISE: A vague feeling of bodily discomfort.

MASTURBATION: Self-stimulation of the genitals for sexual pleasure.

MATURE: Fully developed.

MELANOMA: A malignant tumor arising from melanin (dark pigment) producing systems of the skin.

MENOPAUSE: Cessation of menstruation in the human female; climacteric.

MENSES: The monthly flow of blood from the genital tract of women.

MENSTRUATION: The cyclic, physiological uterine bleeding, which usually occurs at approximately four week intervals, in the absence of pregnancy during the reproductive period of the female; menses.

MIGRAINE: A condition marked by recurrent, severe, vascular (blood vessels) headaches often with nausea and vomiting.

MUCOSAL LINING: Covering of the internal structures that secrete mucus (slime).

MYOCARDIAL INFARCT: Tissue (heart muscle) death due to deprived blood supply by obstruction of an artery by a thrombus (clot).

NEUROLOGICAL: Pertains to the nervous system; the brain, spinal cord and the peripheral nerves.

OBSESSIVE: Pertaining to thought, image or impulse that is unwanted or distressing and comes involuntarily to mind despite attempts to ignore or suppress it.

ORGASM: The climax of sexual excitement marked normally by ejaculation of semen by the male and by the release of tumescence in erectile organs of both sexes.

OSTEOPOROSIS: Abnormal loss of bone tissue, seen most commonly in the elderly.

OVARY: Sexual gland in which the ova (egg) are formed.

OVULATION: The production or discharge of an egg from the ovary in women.

PATHOLOGICAL: Of or concerned with disease; due to or involving disease.

PECTORALS: Pertaining to the chest., e.g., the pectoral muscles.

PELVIC: Pertaining to the lower portion of the trunk, bound by the two hip bones and the sacrum (triangular bone beneath the lumbar vertebrae).

PENILE: Pertaining to the penis, the male organ of copulation and of urinary excretion.

PHARMACOLOGICAL: Pertaining to the science that deals with the effects and uses of drugs.

PHOBIA: Irrational, intense fear of a specific object, activity or situation; a fear that is recognized as excessive or unreasonable by the individual.

PHYSIOLOGIC: Normal, not pathologic; characteristic of conforming to the normal functioning of the body.

PITUITARY: Pertaining to the "master gland" located in the head that affects breast and gonad function.

PMS: Premenstrual syndrome; a syndrome of unknown cause that precedes female menstruation, sometimes marked by bloating, emotional lability, headaches, food cravings, breast swelling and discomfort and decreased ability to concentrate.

PRESBYOPIA: An impairment of vision due to advancing years, causing the near point of distinct vision to be removed farther from the eye.

PROGESTERONE: Hormone produced by the corpus luteum after ovulation in women.

PROSTATE: A gland in the male which surrounds the neck of the bladder and the urethra. The prostate contributes to the semen fluid.

PSYCHE: The human faculty for thought, judgment and

emotion; the mental life, including both conscious and unconscious processes.

PSYCHIATRIST: A physician who specializes in that branch of medicine which deals with the study, treatment and prevention of mental disorders.

PSYCHOGENIC: Having an emotional or psychological origin in reference to symptoms, as opposed to a physiological, or organic basis.

PSYCHOLOGICAL: Pertaining to psychology; derived from the mind or the emotions.

PSYCHOLOGIST: A qualified specialist in that branch of science which deals with the mind and mental processes, especially in relation to human behavior.

PSYCHOSOMATIC: Pertaining to the mind-body relationship; having bodily symptoms of psychic, emotional or mental origins.

QUADRICEPS: The large muscle in the front part of the thigh.

SCROTUM: The pouch which contains the testes.

SEDATIVE: A drug or other agent that allays excitement.

SEMEN: (seminal fluid): The thick, whitish secretion of the reproductive organs in the male; composed of sperm, secretions from the prostate, seminal vesicles and various other glands.

SEXUALITY: The characteristic quality of the male and female reproductive elements; the constitution of an individual in relation to sexual attitudes or activity.

STEROID: A group name for compounds that have similar chemical characteristics; in this group are progesterone, adrenal hormones, the gonadal hormones (including testosterone), and cholesterol.

STRESS: The sum of all nonspecific biological reactions to any adverse stimulus, physical, mental or emotional, internal or external, that tends to disturb the organism's homeostasis (a tendency to stability in the normal body states): should these compensating reactions be inadequate or inappropriate, they may lead to disorders. The term is also used to refer to the stimuli that elicit that reactions; forcibly exerted influence or pressure.

STRESSORS: Adverse internal or external influences.

SYMPTOM: Any subjective evidence of disease or of a patient's condition; such evidence as perceived by the patient; a change in a patient's condition indicative of some bodily or mental state.

SYNDROME: A set of symptoms which occur together; the sum of signs of any abnormal state; a symptom complex.

TESTES: Plural of testis, the male gonads normally situated in the scrotum.

TESTOSTERONE: The hormone produced by cells of the testes which functions in the induction and maintenance of male secondary sex characteristics.

THERAPEUTIC: Pertaining to the art of healing; curative.

THERAPIST: A person skilled in the treatment of disease.

TRANQUILIZER: A drug or other agent which works on the emotional state, quieting or calming the patient without affecting clarity of consciousness.

TRAUMA: Injury whether physical or psychic.

TRIGLYCERIDES: Compounds consisting of three molecules of fatty acid. It is a fat synthesized from carbohydrates for storage in fat cells.

TUMESCENCE: The condition of being swollen; a swollen organ.

VAGINAL: Pertaining to the vagina, the passage leading from the external genital orifice to the uterus in women.

VIRILITY: Masculine vigor, potency, or passion; manliness.

Suggested Readings

Amodeo, John and Kris. *Being Intimate: A Guide to Successful Relationships*. New York: Arkana Paperbacks, 1986.

Barbach, Lonnie G., and David L. Geisinger. *Going the Distance: Secrets to Lifelong Love*. New York: Doubleday, 1991.

Bolen, Jean Shinada. *Gods in Everyman: A New Psychology of Men's Lives and Loves*. San Francisco: Harper & Row, 1992.

Bowskill, Derek, and Anthea Linacre. *The Male Menopause*. California: Brooke House, 1977.

Brecher, Edward M. *Love, Sex & Aging*. Boston/Toronto: Little, Brown, 1984.

Bridges, William. *Transitions: Making Sense of Life's Changes*. New York: Addison-Wesley, 1980.

Burns, David D. *Feeling Good: The New Mood Therapy*. New York: Morrow, 1980.

Castleman, Michael. *Sexual Solutions*. New York: Simon and Schuster, 1980.

Feinstein, David, and Peg Elliott Mayo. *Rituals for Living and Dying*. San Francisco: HarperSanFrancisco, 1990.

Gilbaugh, James H. *A Doctor's Guide to Men's Private Parts*. New York: Crown, 1989.

Glassner, Barry. *Bodies: Why We Look the Way We Do*. New York: Putnam, 1988.

Goin, John M., and Marcia Kraft Goin. *Changing the Body: Psychological Effects of Plastic Surgery*. Baltimore: Williams and Wilkins, 1981.

Hostility, Coping and Health. Washington, D.C: American Psychological Association, 1992.

Johnson, Robert A. *He: Understanding Masculine Psychology*. New York: Harper and Row, 1977, 1989.

Johnson, Robert A. *She: Understanding Feminine Psychology*. New York: Harper and Row, 1977, 1989.

Johnson, Robert A. *We: Understanding the Psychology of Romantic Love*. New York: Harper and Row, 1983.

Kübler-Ross, Elizabeth. *Death, The Final Stages of Growth*. Englewood Cliffs, New Jersey: Prentice-Hall, 1975.

Levinson, Daniel J. et. al *The Seasons of a Man's Life*. New York: Knopf, 1978.

Liebman, Joshua Loth. *Peace of Mind*. New York: Simon and Schuster, 1946.

Masters, William M., and Virginia E. Johnson. *Human Sexual Inadequacy*. Boston: Little Brown, 1970; New York: Bantam, 1980.

Mayer, Mancy. *The Male Mid-life Crisis*. New York: NAL, 1970, Signet, 1978.

Moog, Carol. *Are They Selling Her Lips: Advertising and Identity*. New York: William Morrow, 1990.

Moore, Robert L., and Douglas Gillette. *King, Warrior, Magician, Lover*. San Francisco: HarperSanFrancisco, 1990.

Morganstern, Steven, and Allen E. Abrahams. *Love Again, Live Again*. Englewood Cliffs, New Jersey: Prentice Hall, 1988.

Ruebsaat,, Helmut J., M.D., and Raymond Hull. *The Male Climacteric*. Toronto: Hawthorn Books, 1975.

Schover, Leslie R., and Søren Buus Jensen. *Sexuality and Chronic Illness*. New York: Guilford Press, 1988.

Shapiro, Joan. *Men: A Translation for Women*. New York: Dutton, 1992.

Sheehy, Gail. *The Silent Passage: Menopause*. New York: Random House, 1991.

Stoppard, Miriam. *50-Plus Life Guide*. London: Dorling Kindersley, 1983.

Wholey, Dennis. *Are You Happy?* Boston: Houghton Mifflin, 1986.

Selected Bibliography

Adrenal Secretions of Male and Female Hormones

Baird, D.T., A. Uno, and J. Melby. 1969. Adrenal secretion of androgens and estrogens. *J. Endocrinology.* 45:135-136.

Regno, F.D. 1975. Andropause and its treatment. *Clinical Ter.* 75:219.

Vermeulen, A. 1980. Adrenal androgens and aging. *Adrenal Androgens.* 207.

Andropause as a Psychological Condition

Aquilina, R.G. 1984. *How to survive the male menopause.* London: Elm Tree Books.

Bowskill, D., and A. Linacre. 1976. *The "Male" menopause.* London: Frederick Muller.

Datan, N., and D. Rodeheaver. 1983. *Beyond gennativity: Toward a sensuality of later life.* In *Sexuality in later years,* edited by R.B. Weg, 179-288. New York/London: Academic Press.

Featherstone, M., and M. Hepworth. 1985. The male menopause: Lifestyle and sexuality. *Maturitas.* 7:235-246.

Rosenberg, S.D., and M.P. Farrell. 1976. Identity crisis in

middle-aged men. *Intl. J. Aging and Human Development.* 7:153-170.

Comparing Male and Female Menopause

Jaszmann, L. 1978. *De middelbare leeftijd van de man.* Deventer, Netherlands: Van Loghum Slaterus.

Kupperman, H.S. 1974. Treating menopausal women and climacteric men. *Medical World News.* 15:32.

van Keep, P.A., D.M. Serr, and R.B. Greenblatt, eds. 1979. *Female and male climacteric.* London: MTP Press.

Defining Andropause

Rubens, R. 1987. "Historical overview of the concept of andropause." Paper read at Proceedings of the Fifth Intl. Congress on the Menopause, Sorrento, Italy, April 6-8.

Rubens, R. 1987. Interview with author. Sorrento, Italy, 8 April.

Early Research in Male Menopause

Werner, A.A. 1939. The male climacteric. *JAMA.* 112:1341.

Erectile Dysfunction

Burnett, C. 1992. Nitric oxide: A physiologic mediator of penile erection. *Science.* 257:401-403.

Drugs that cause sexual dysfunction. 1987. *The Medical Letter on Drugs & Therapeutics.* 29:65.

Krone, R.J. 1989. Impotence. *New Eng. J. of Medicine.* 32:1648.

Morley, J.E. 1986. Impotence. *Amer. J. Medicine.* 80:897-905.

Whitehead, E.D. 1990. Diagnostic evaluation of impotence. *Post. Graduate Medicine.* 88:123.

Sex and the Male Menopause

Featherstone, M., and M. Hepworth. 1985. The history of the

male menopause. *Maturitas.* 7:249-257.

Kinsey, A.C. 1948. *Sexual behavior in the human male.* Philadelphia/London: W.B Saunders Co.

Livson, F.B. 1983. Gender identity: *A life-span view of sex role development.* In *Sexuality in later years,* edited by R.B. Weg. New York/London: Academic Press.

Masters, W.H., and V.E. Johnson. 1966. *Sexual Aging: Human sexual responses.* Boston: Little Brown.

Gadpaille, W.J., and Lief, H.I., eds 1981. *Sexual problems in medical practice.* American Medical Assoc.

Terminology: Andropause

Flint, M. 1979. Culture and the climacteric. *J. of Biosocial Science.* 6:197.

Gooren, L., and R. Rubens. 1987. *Overview of the concept of the andropause.* In *The climacteric and beyond,* edited by L. Zichella, D.M. Whitehead, and P.A. van Keep, 85-93. New Jersey: Parthenon Publishing Group.

Terminology: Viropause

Sheehy, G. The unspeakable passage: Is there a male menopause? *Vanity Fair.*

Testosterone Deficiency

Aagoord, T.L 1989. Erogenic drugs. *Audio Digest.* 37:38.

Feldman, J.M., R.W. Postlethwaite, and J.F. Glenn. 1976. Hot flashes and sweats in men with testicular insufficiency. *Archives of Internal Medicine.* 136:606.

Horton R., P. Hsieh, J. Barberia, L. Pages, and M. Cosgrove. 1975. Altered blood androgens in elderly men with benign prostatic hyperplasia. *J. Clinical Edocrinology and Metabolism.* 41:793.

Korenman, S.G. 1990. Secondary hypogonadism in older men:

Its relationship to impotence. *J. Clincal Endocrinology and Metabolism.* 71:963.

Korenman, S.G. 1990. Use of a vacuum tumescence device in the management of impotence. *J. Amer. Geriatric Society.* 38:217.

Lynch, J.M. 1991. Use and abuse of anabolic steroids. *Audio Digest., Family Practice.* 39:34.

Morley, J.E. 1989. Sexual function with advancing age. *Medical Clinics of North America.* 73:1483-1496.

Persky, H., C.P. O'Brien, E. Fine, W.J. Howard, M.A. Khan, and R.W. Beck. 1977. The effect of alcohol and smoking on testosterone function and aggression in chronic alcoholics. *Am. J. Psychiatry.* 134:621-625.

Sandeman, T.F. 1975. The possible dangers of androgens used for male climacteric. *Medical J. Aust.* 1:634-635.

Sarfaty, C. 1972. The use of androgens in the male climacteric. *Medical J. Aust.* 2:571.

Serio, M., P. Gonnelli, D. Borrelli, A. Pampaloni, G. Fiorelli, E. Calabresi, G. Forti, M. Pazzagli, M. Mannelli, A. Baroni, P. Giannotti, and G. Giusti. 1979. Human testicular secretion with increasing age. *J. Steroid Biochemistry.* 11:893-897.

Spark, R.F. 1983. Neuroendocrinology and impotence. *Annual Internal Medicine.* 98:103.

Sparrow, D., R. Bosse, and J.W. Rowe. 1980. The influence of age, alcohol consumption, and body building on gonadal function in men. *J. Clinical Endocrinal Metabolism* 51:508.

Tsitouras, P.D., C.E. Martin, and M. Harman. 1982. Relationship of serum testosterone to sexual activity in healthy elderly men. *J. Gerontology.* 37:288.